ARTS, CRAFTS AND TRADITIONAL INDUSTRIES

(Book 1)

DR. ASIM K. DASGUPTA

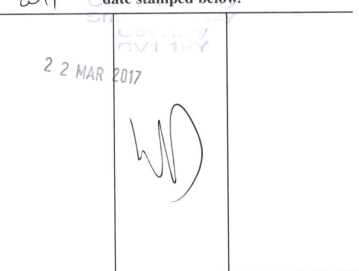

AuthorHouse™ UK Ltd.
500 Avebury Boulevard
Central Milton Keynes, MK9 2BE
www.authorhouse.co.uk
Phone: 08001974150

First published by AuthorHouse November 2011
Reprinted by AuthorHouse April 2012

ISBN: 978-1-4567-9233-6 (sc)

This book is printed on acid-free paper.

authorHOUSE®

About the Author

DR. ASIM K. DASGUPTA is an occupational physician who retired as a Consultant from the National Health Service in United Kingdom and also worked in small, medium and large or heavy industries. His work, research and interests have taken him to various countries of the world which has helped him to write this book. His training, qualifications, teaching, experiences and hobbies have also played an important role in writing this craft book. He is a medical graduate from Calcutta University and has got a postgraduate degree (MSc.) from London University. He has also obtained a Diploma in Tropical Medicine & Hygiene from Liverpool University and a Diploma in Industrial Health, from the Royal College of Physicians and Surgeons, England. He is a Member of the Faculty of Occupational Medicine (MFOM), London and a Member of the Royal College of Physicians, London. He has also written a book, entitled 'Disasters' whose second edition has been recently published. He lives in Hampshire, United Kingdom.

From the Kirkus Indie Review Feb. 16th, 2012

A thorough guide best suited for people working in or responsible for safety and health aspects of these industries, or as a starting point for those wanting to learn more.

In the first of five books in a planned series Dr Dasgupta uses first hand accounts to provide an overview of traditional craft industries.

The descriptions of the cultural aspects are a strength of the book, as Dasgupta emphasizes how developing countries still depend heavily on handmade goods, providing the reader with an understanding of the important role carried out by people who continue to work in handmade and traditional craft industries at a time when other industries are dominating the marketplace.

Using an encyclopedia format, Dasgupta (Disasters, 2011) describes typical crafts, such as sewing and basket weaving, but also stretches the definition of "craft" with entries such as lavender harvesting. The entries, which are randomly presented, fall into three general areas: decorative jewellery, clothing and housewares (embroidery, bangle-making and glass-making); harvesting of crops (sugar cane, coffee, tea); and industrial goods (plastics, rope-making and brick-making). Each chapter follows a similar structure and format, starting with historic origins of the craft, followed by a list of products and chemicals used, the cultural and social impact of each industry and a list of health and safety hazards. Large colour photos also depict activities involved in the practice of the craft.

Contents

Preface

From ancient times the human race has shown an interest in arts and crafts, and artisans have been discovering and displaying their skills through invention. Civilisation flourishes thanks to their contributions, and their countries get richer from the import and export of their products.
Some products are the traditional arts and crafts of local areas which largely depend upon locally available materials. Many arts and crafts industries are family traditions or family businesses, and the skills are passed down from generation to generation. Family-oriented handicraft businesses and traditional arts and crafts became industries as the demand for machine-made factory goods increased. However, globalisation and cheap mass production were bound to have an impact on the survival of certain traditional types of arts and crafts. This means that some traditional hand-made arts and crafts are gradually dying out throughout the world, although some of the poor and developing countries or underdeveloped regions of the world still rely on traditional hand-made products.

In five books I have tried to describe about 100 traditional arts and crafts or industries: their history, invention, materials, geographical locations and methods of making products. Lastly exposure or handling-related health issues or hazards during the manufacturing process are outlined so that handlers and manufactures can be aware of the health issues. I have written these books from the experiences that I have gained while working, researching, travelling and visiting industries, plantations, arts, crafts and handicrafts centres, museums, markets and shops throughout the world. From the raw materials in remote places (including agricultural origins) to the finished products selling on the markets, I have observed their various processes. I have recorded, photographed and collected materials over the years and am now producing them in book form. This is the first book, where I have described 20 crafts; the rest will appear gradually in a series of four books. This book is written to be accessible to the general public, manufacturers, apprentices, arts and crafts students and also others who are interested in undertaking, or taking up as a hobby, these listed arts and crafts. The book will also be helpful to healthcare workers and professionals as well as others who are involved in ensuring the health, safety and wellbeing of all persons in these arts and crafts businesses. This is specially for occupational physicians and general practitioners who are interested in knowing the processes and exposure related health issues.

Chapter 1: Bangles

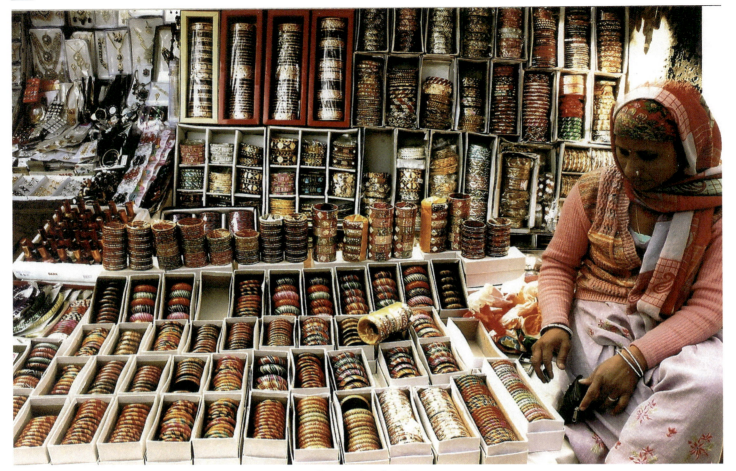

Bangle Seller

Bangles are traditional ornaments usually worn by women and girls in South Asia. They are usually worn in pairs, one or more on either wrists or arms. They are circular in shape and made from glass, shell, copper, bronze, gold, silver, lacquer (a resinous substance deposited by the lacquer insect on trees), bone, wood, horn, acrylic, crystal, plastic, steel or other metals such as aluminium or platinum. Sometimes men wear a single bangle on the wrist or arm.

The excavation of multiple archaeological sites in South Asia supports the idea that bangle wearing is an ancient art in the Indian subcontinent. A statuette excavated from a site of the Mohenjo-Daro civilisation (2600 BC) shows a dancing girl wearing bangles on her left arm. Copper, gold and shell bangles have been discovered on various other excavated sites belonging to the Mauryan period (322-185 BC).
The ancient Egyptians made glass ornaments by using soda (Na_2CO_3) together with other ingredients.

The process of glass bangle-making involves various stages. Raw glass is made in the furnace at a temperature of about 1400°C by mixing primarily soda ash, silica (sand) and other additives. The molten glass is drawn out from the furnace with the pipes in the form of a globule and is transferred to another furnace where the formation of spirals from the molten glass takes place with the help of a mounted spindle that is rotated manually. The size of the bangles mainly depends on the diameter of the spindle used in the formation of these spirals. The spirals are taken off the spindle and cut in order to make the bangles.

The cut bangles are then sent to have the ends joined; this is done by heating the ends in an ordinary chimney fired by coal, kerosene oil or gas connected to a simple hand-made air compressor for air input. The joined bangles then go for finishing, colouring, designing, polishing and decorating. Designing is done on a grinding wheel operated by an electric motor. A special type of polishing is completed with synthetic or pure gold. For decorating and colouring the bangles, resins, hardener and salts of various metals such as arsenic, lead, zinc, copper, manganese, cobalt, cadmium, selenium are usually used. The finishing process ends with the sorting and packaging of the bangles.

Although bangles are seen in many parts of the world, India and Pakistan are the traditional bangle-making countries. Colourful glass bangles are mostly produced in Firozabad in India and Hyderabad in Pakistan. The coloured multiple bangles worn by Indian women at weddings and other festivals attach interesting meanings and symbolism to the various colours. Red colour means energy and love; blue is for tranquillity and wisdom; purple is for independence; green is for luck; orange is for success; yellow is for happiness; white is for new beginnings and purity; black is for power and strength. A gold or gold-coloured bangle symbolises fortune. Silver or silver colour symbolises strength and purity.

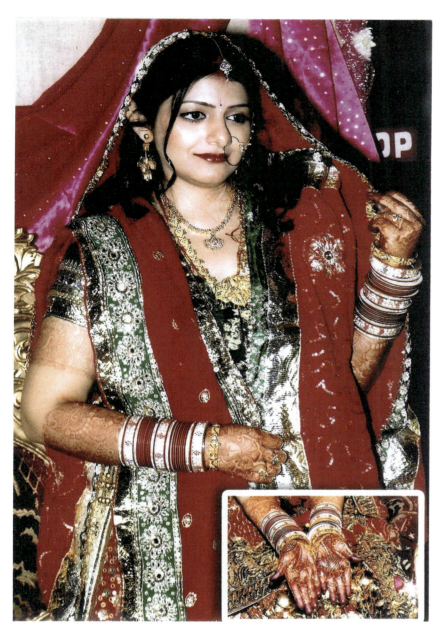

Indian bride wearing colourful bangles

WHAT ARE THE HEALTH ISSUES?

The bangle-making industry in India and Pakistan employs not only men and women but also boys and girls. Health risks arise from working in the proximity of the furnaces used in moulding and joining processes, as well as from toxic chemicals during coating and painting. The main physical hazards are accidents from fire and splash burns to the skin; injuries from molten glass while carrying; injuries from the use of heavy and sharp tools; and thermal stress. Respiratory diseases and musculo-skeletal disorders have also been reported. Metal-and lacquer-related respiratory impairments include asthma, feelings of suffocation, and nasal, throat and eye irritations which are directly related to the duration of exposure.

Chapter 2: Basket Making

Basket making is a kind of weaving process whereby vegetable fibres are used without spinning. The materials are willow, cane, bamboo, reeds, local grasses and plants, coconut, date and palm leaves. The fibrous materials are usually bent and shaped to form a basket. Most baskets consist of three main parts: the base, the side walls and the rim. Some baskets have a lid or handle. Baskets can be of various sizes, shapes, patterns, styles or colours. The basket-making process has its own terminology: static, spokes, stakes etc. 'Static' refers to the pieces of work materials which are laid down first. 'Spokes' relate to round baskets; for other shapes of baskets they are usually called 'stakes'. Whatever the shape, the weaver fills in the sides of the basket by hand weaving. The weavers who make the baskets are usually called 'basket makers' and the tools they use are machetes, knives, reed cutters, scissors, secateurs, tallow, traditional cow horn, raping irons, shavers, cleavers, wooden-handled bodkins, etc.

Basket making is an ancient art and its history goes back alongside the history of human evolution. The oldest known basket is 10,000-12,000 years old (carbon dated) and was found in Upper Egypt.

Willow is the basket-making plant which grows in the northern hemisphere. The tree concerned is from the genus *salix*, which grows in cold, moist environments and needs plenty of water. Hence they are found in both cold and temperate regions of the northern hemisphere along the banks of rivers and marshes. In Britain the main willow-growing areas are Somerset and Devon (around Exeter), where English willow baskets are made.

Willow harvesting takes place annually. Herbicides, pesticides and insecticides are used to control weeds, pest and disease during willow cultivation. Cutting takes place in winter. Once the willow twigs are cut, they undergo various processes such as sorting, boiling, peeling, stripping (by hand or machine), drying and tying before the willow-basket maker makes the basket.

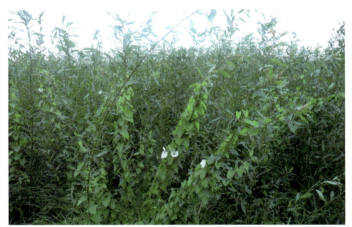

Willow growing in South-West England

The willow-basket makers follow certain patterns in their work: *bordering* (weaving around the top of the basket), *fitching* (open-work weaving with parallel or criss-cross rods), *randing* (where weaving is done using single strands of willow), *slewing* (where weaving is done using multiple strands of willow), and *waling* (weaving around the base of the basket for extra strength and shape).

Basket weaving

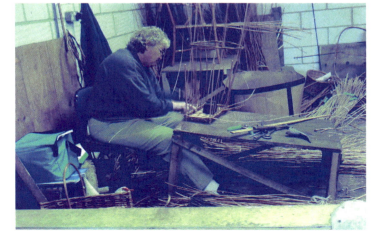

Cane and bamboo are natural products which grow abundantly in India, Bangladesh, Burma, Thailand, Sri Lanka and other South-East Asian countries as well as the southern USA. The high tensile strength of the bamboo and cane makes them easy to mould into various shapes and forms.

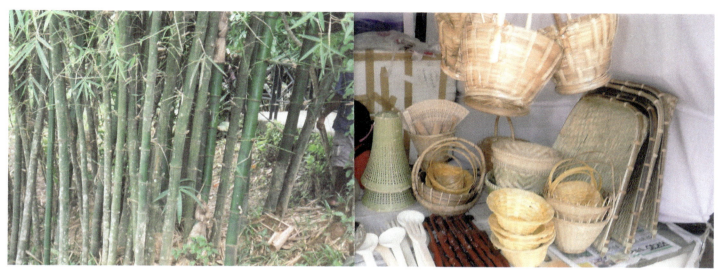

Bamboo grove and Bamboo-baskets

The cane is sometimes heated and bent over a charcoal fire and then coiled together; the coil is smoked carefully to make it insect- as well as water-proof. Prior to basket making, the canes are usually soaked for 24 hours in clean water, then cut into strips and dyed. Canes and bamboo for basket making have to be even: this is ensured by splitting them vertically into very fine uniform strips and then cutting to the preferred length (spoke) using a knife or scissors. Sometimes they are dyed or bleached. Whether dyed or natural they are usually kept in cool dry place to prevent mould growing on the coils.

Native Americans in the USA and people in some other regions of the world make baskets from locally available grasses, roots, bark and other plants. The basket makers gather the materials, which are usually sprayed with pesticides and are therefore toxic. They use dyes from flowers. They peel the bark with their teeth, moisten the ends of sticks with their tongues, and hold materials in their mouths while making baskets. Basket making from coconut, date or palm leaves is common where these trees are grown – typically in the tropical, subtropical and warm temperate climate regions of the world. In India, coconut and palm leaves are woven into a basket to be used to draw water. In Oman and some other Arab countries, baskets are made from date and palm leaves which are wide and ribbon like. The fronds are cut from trees and collected, and then the leaves are removed by steam and put in water to make them flexible and produce strong long bands. They are kept in store until the actual weaving process commences, using these long bands. In the final stage of weaving the rolls of bands are again put in water.

WHAT ARE THE HEALTH ISSUES?

Finger injuries, repetitive strain injuries, musculo-skeletal and skin disorders have been reported among basket makers. Tool- and strip- related accidental injuries can occur. Burns and dye-related health issues are also there. Exposure to toxic pesticides and herbicides can increase the risk of certain cancers (mouth, skin, breast), allergies, rashes, breathing difficulties, flu-like illnesses, nausea, dizziness, respiratory disorders and neuropathy.

Chapter 3: Brass and Metal Working

Brass making is a form of metal working; brass is an alloy of copper and zinc. Similarly, bronze is an alloy of copper and tin. Although metal was used in Palaeolithic times (the Old Stone Age) and the Copper Age, advanced metal working did not occur until the Bronze Age, and this was the age when heavy metal usage began. In this prehistoric society, smelting copper and tin from naturally occurring outcrop of copper and tin ores, creating a bronze alloy by melting those metals together and casting them into bronze artefacts, constituted the art of metallurgy. Metallurgy is commonly used as part of the craft of metal making. The art was most probably invented as far back as the fourth millennium BC.

More than 15,000 years ago, Egyptians used copper for their utensils, weapons and ornaments. By 4000 BC, the knowledge of metal making had spread to Europe. India is well known for the making of brass and copper objects. The history of metal making in South Asia goes back beyond the Indus Valley Civilisation and the inhabitants of the ancient Indus Valley; the Harappans developed techniques in metallurgy and produced copper, bronze, lead and tin.

India is the largest brass-making country in the world: places like Moradabad, Varanasi, Mirzapur in Uttar Pradesh, Rajasthan, West Bengal, Orissa, Madhya Pradesh, Andhra Pradesh, and Ladakh make up the brass-making region of India. India's famous metal-casting techniques include *bidri* work (silver and brass inlaid upon zinc and copper which are blackened using a solution of copper sulphate) in Karnataka; *dokra* work (which is a 'wax process' of metal casting with brass scraps used as raw materials) in West Bengal; and *filigree* art (fine silver thread work) in Orissa. Tamil Nadu and Kerala, in South India, are renowned for their variety of special lamps made of copper and brass, which are very ancient and traditional local arts. The most famous brass and copper crafts in India are brassware, copperware, utensils, idols, deities, bronze figures, statues (including animals), lamps, vases, bowls, caskets, picture frames, planters and brass stoves.

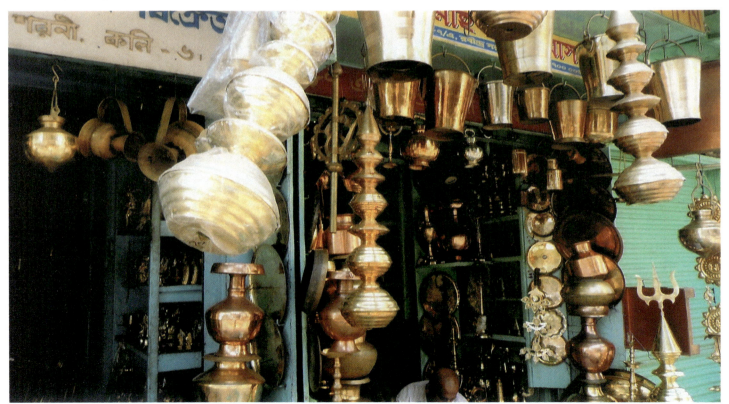

Copper and brass products

Brass sheets are primarily made from the alloys. In their turn, the alloys for brass sheets are generally made by combining the constituent elements, copper and zinc, into a melt (liquid state). The melt is then solidified into an ingot or is poured into a near-net-shape (as in a cast). The transformation from ingot to final sheet requires a process of mechanical reduction such as rolling. The rolling can be either cold (rolling at room temperature) or hot (hot rolling). The process can be continuous, i.e. from melt to solid form and then rolling into the sheet.

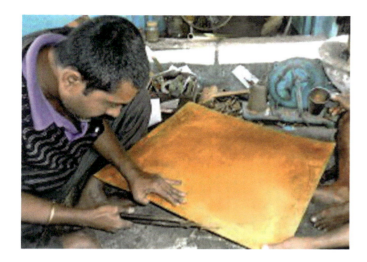

Brass sheet cutting by hand

For moulding, some small-scale industries use an underground furnace that is fanned by rotating wheels. The ingot is put on the top of the furnace and broken into small pieces with a hammer; the worker then melts the required amount of brass. The molten brass along with other raw materials is poured into a graphite crucible held between long tongs.

In this process everything is done manually and the task involves a) rotating the fan, b) pouring the brass into moulds, c) removing the crucible, and d) replacing it in the furnace at a temperature of 1100°C.

However, brass or any metal making comes down to a technique by which the metals are shaped by processes such as casting, moulding, polishing, scraping, welding, grinding, colouring and engraving.

Brassware engraving

WHAT ARE THE HEALTH ISSUES?

In the metal-working industry in India not only men, but also women and children are employed and poor working and living conditions have been found. Moreover, tuberculosis and short life span amongst children working in brassware industries have also been reported. Injuries are common and these can occur while handling, lifting or carrying, or from slipping, tripping or falling or being hit by moving, flying or falling objects. Molten-metal-related burns can occur. Adverse health effects take the form of skin diseases, respiratory diseases (occupational asthma, chronic bronchitis) and musculo-skeletal disorders.

Chapter 4: Brick Making

Bricks always go with the construction industry and are the commonest and most essential of building materials. Bricks are usually made from certain types of clay, which is pressed and shaped into the blocks and then fired into hardness in a kiln. At first brick making was manual: clay was moulded and dried in the sun. Bricks are usually made close to a suitable supply of clay, usually a river bed or clay pits.

The history of brick making goes back approximately 5000 years in the Tigris-Euphrates basin: the ancient human race in that area was probably the first ever to use bricks. In Babylonia, brick makers relied on the thick clay deposited by the overflowing river as the only material available to them for construction of buildings. Persians and Assyrians used sun-dried blocks of clay, whereas Egyptians and Greeks used bricks only to a limited extent, preferring marble and stone which were available to them in plenty. Romans used bricks extensively and gave an important role to fired bricks as basic structural materials in the construction of buildings throughout the Roman Empire. The old method of making brick was replaced by a mechanical method at the beginning of the nineteenth century. Clay for brick making is taken from river beds or shovelled from pits.

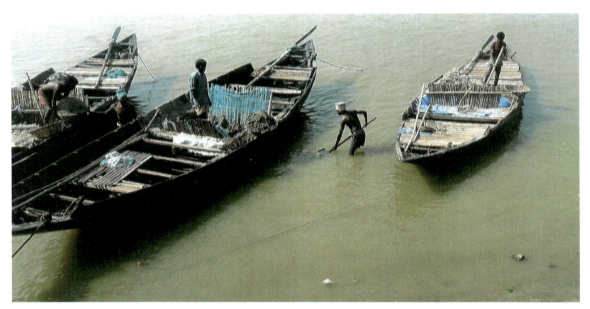

Clay extraction from the river bed

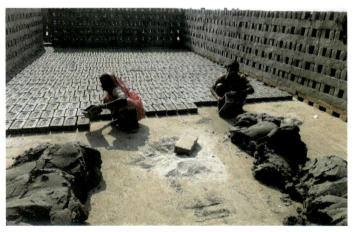

***Clay mould and hand-made bricks
before firing***

The raw clay is crushed into fine particles and sieved. Then it is mixed with water to produce a doughy mass; this type of softening can be done either by hand or by machine. The clay mould, made by hand, is coated with sand. For machine-moulded bricks, clay is mixed with additives such as colorants and sand. In the brick-making machine the clay is pressed out through a rectangular hole in the form of blocks which are sliced into individual bricks by the cutting machine. Then they go for firing.

Before firing the bricks are usually dried in hot air and cooled. Firing usually takes place in a brick kiln at a temperature between 800°and 1100°C depending on the type of clay used. The clay and sand used for bricks contain free silica.

Besides clay bricks, there are other types such as concrete bricks, ash-clay bricks, fire bricks, coloured bricks and special shaped bricks.
Concrete bricks are made from crushed limestone or granite bonded with cement and coloured with pigments such as iron oxides. Mechanical or hydraulic presses are used to make these kinds of bricks. Ash-clay bricks are made from a combination of ash (solid waste from coal-fired power plants) and local clay which are hydraulically pressed and fixed at a temperature of 1000°C. Fire bricks are heat-resistant bricks which are made of special refractory materials called fire clays, and are fixed at a very high temperature.

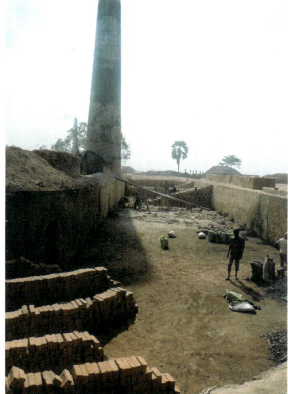
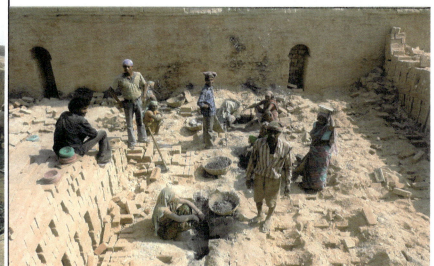

Brick kiln and bricks after firing

Currently China and India are the two top brick-making countries. In some countries in Africa, Asia and Latin America, women and children are employed.

WHAT ARE THE HEALTH ISSUES?

Injuries while handling, lifting or carrying, or from slipping, tripping, falling or being hit by moving, flying or falling objects have been reported. Burn injuries can also occur. Silicosis, Chronic Obstructive Pulmonary Disease (COPD), lung cancer, tuberculosis and musculo-skeletal disorders are the ill-health issues in brick-making industries.

Chapter 5: Carpet Making

A carpet is a kind of textile covering and is usually produced on a loom, similar to woven cloth. Carpets which are used for floor covering are known as floor carpets or runners. Wall and table coverings are called wall and table carpets. The most richly decorated carpets are called felt rugs. Fibres and yarns used in carpets include wool, wool blended with synthetic fibres, silk, nylon, polypropylene, polyester, polymer and so on. Cotton and jute are used for binding and for weft respectively. There are three types of carpet use: a) religious, social or ceremonial functions; b) artistic, such as bolsters embroidered with gold and silk thread; and c) home, office or commercial premises furnishing (both decorative and utility). The fitting of carpets in homes, public buildings, hotels, shops and offices is mainly for thermal and acoustic reasons.

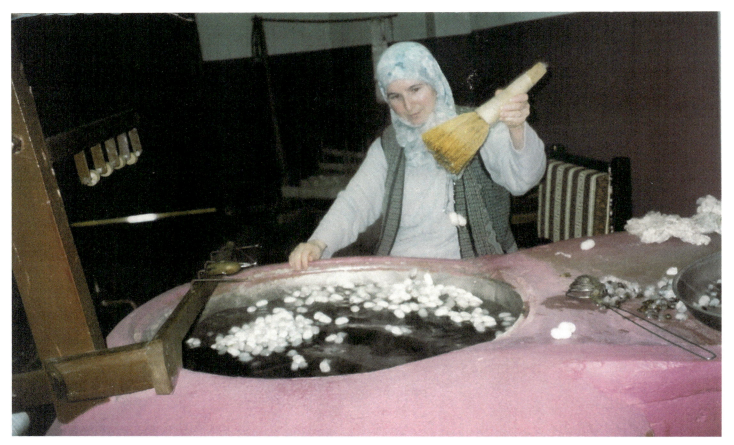

Woman spinning silk threads from cocoons for Turkish carpets

Historically, the carpet-producing regions of the world are Turkey, Persia (Iran), Turkestan, the Caucasus, Afghanistan, Pakistan, India, Nepal and China. For centuries women played the main role in carpet making, and this creative art is passed from generation to generation, especially if it is a family-oriented handicrafts business. In some societies, a daughter would have a greater chance of marrying if she was a skilled weaver and could offer carpets as part of a dowry to her future husband.

Although traditionally women are employed in the carpet industry, children are also used in some carpet-making countries like India, Pakistan and Nepal. The manufacturers claim that the nimble fingers of children are essential to form the intricate designs used in the carpet, but many people disagree with this. Most probably the children are employed because they can be made to accept low wages and poor working conditions.

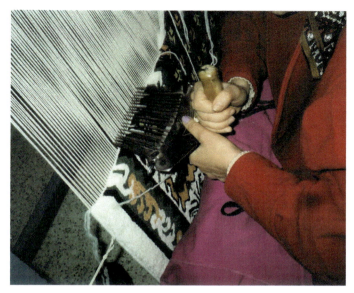

Carpet weaver (Tunisia)

Carpets were probably first made by nomadic peoples in Central Asia and there is evidence from c. 6000 BC of goats and sheep being sheared for wool and hair, which was then spun and woven. The Egyptian, Chinese and Mayan civilisations knew the carpet-making art. An archaeological discovery in the Pazyrak valley among the Altai Mountains in Siberia was the first evidence of a 'hand knotted' carpet that was 2400 to 2500 years old. The first documented evidence of the existence of carpets was found in a Chinese textbook dating back to 224-641 AD, although there is written evidence of rug weaving, in Nepal and India in the second century AD. In the eighth to tenth centuries, various decorative carpets were used as furnishings, indicative of social status in the Near and Middle East.

The manufacturing of carpets with coloured fabrics and embroidered patterns using silk and wool expanded with conquest and the migration of craftsmen and artisans in Central Asia, Persia and Turkey. Some of the greatest carpet-making centres developed in Persia and Turkey. In the fifteenth to sixteenth centuries an interest in oriental rugs and carpets appeared in the courts of Europe. After that many Europeans showed their enthusiasm for carpets, and Americans followed suit. Industrial development in England in the seventeenth and eighteenth centuries had a great impact on carpet making: it started to be done in the western world instead of importing carpets from the east. Machine-made carpet factories started to appear in Scotland, England and the USA. In the mid-nineteenth century tufted carpets developed in the USA; by the end of that century woven carpet production had declined and production of tufted carpet had increased. Developments in man-made fibres, loom widths and machine efficiencies brought carpets within the reach of the mass market.

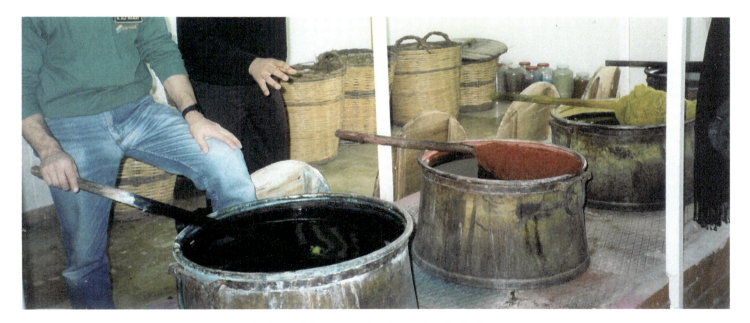

Bleaching and chemical dying

14 However, the art of traditional carpet making or weaving, which requires a loom, wool and basic weaving tools, cannot be replaced by machines although machine-made carpet benefits from mass production and common utilisation. The demand for hand-made carpets will be there as long as the rich colours, varied patterns and quality of design of carpets persist and hand-made carpet producing countries can hold on in today's competitive global market. In the process thread making, dye making (mixing and colouring the textile fibres), designing, and finally weaving all have important role in carpet making. While weaving carpets, wrist and finger flexions and extensions are used repeatedly, along with pinching movements and firm grasping.

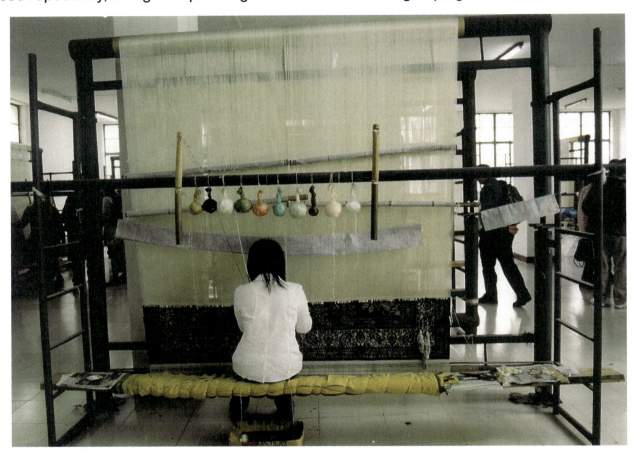

Artistic carpet weaving with silk threads (China)

WHAT ARE THE HEALTH ISSUES?

Traditionally certain occupations, such as wool weaving, run the risk of respiratory disorders; spinners have been known to suffer from musculo-skeletal disorders. A health survey of the children working in the carpet industry in India showed some evidence of finger deformity, retarded growth, defective vision and respiratory disorders. However, the main ill health issues in carpet industry are: a) posture- and weaving-tool-related musculo-skeletal disorders and injuries. Soft tissues, joints, median nerve (carpal tunnel), back and skin (hyperkeratosis nodules and plaques) are involved. b) dermatitis due to handling of decomposition products of a parasite in the cocoon,c) dust-related respiratory disorders such as chronic bronchitis, chronic obstructive airways diseases (COPD), occupational asthma and pneumonitis, and d) Chemical-dye and bleach-related allergic skin diseases, respiratory irritation and certain cancers (lymphocytic leukaemia and testicular cancer).

Coffee is the most widely used beverage in the world. As coffee drinking rose in popularity, coffee houses sprang up and became the meeting places of intellectuals, politicians and various other groups. Some coffee houses became famous for their social and business activities or connections with romanticism or revolutionary ideas.

Ethiopia is believed to be the birth-place of coffee, as it was the ancestors of the Ethiopians who were the first to discover coffee beans in the hills and formerly wide forests of Ethiopia. It was in the ninth centaury that coffee was discovered in Ethiopia; it then spread to Yemen and Egypt. In the fifteenth century, it was in Sufi monasteries of Yemen that coffee beans were first roasted and brewed in a similar way to that currently practised. In the sixteenth century coffee spread to the Middle East, Persia, Turkey and North Africa. The Ottoman Turks played an important part in spreading coffee throughout their empire. Then it gradually spread to India, Italy, the Netherlands and rest of Europe, Indonesia and America. Currently the coffee-growing countries are Brazil, Colombia, Costa Rica, Ecuador, El Salvador, Ethiopia, Guatemala, Haiti, India, Indonesia, Jamaica, Java, Papua New Guinea, Peru, Uganda, Kenya, Laos, Mexico, USA, Vietnam and Yemen. 90% of the world's coffee is produced in the developing world.

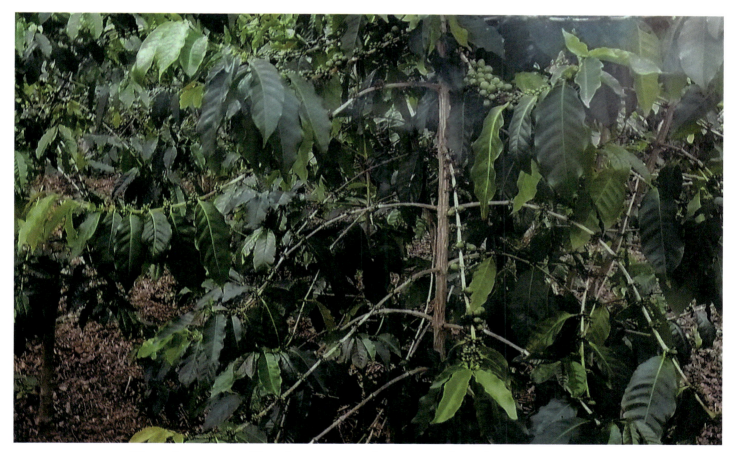

Cherries on coffee trees growing on volcanic soil in Hawaii

A tropical climate is ideal for coffee to grow and coffee trees are usually planted in plantations with high air humidity and an average temperature of at least 20°C. A coffee plant usually starts to produce flowers 3-4 years after being planted, and from the flowers the coffee cherries appear.

16 Ideally the first harvest should be at least 5 years after planting. The trees are usually kept for 25 years and during that period they may bloom every season. The cherries usually ripen eight months after emerging from the flowers, changing colour from green to red. At that point they are harvested.

Coffee is normally harvested during the dry season, being at its best in April and October when the coffee cherries are bright red, glossy and firm enough. Ripe cherries can either be picked by hand or stripped from the trees – along with unripe and overripe cherries – using a harvesting machine. Once the harvesting has been done, manually or by machine, the drying and sorting of the dark red, ripe cherries takes place. Afterwards the coffee beans are separated from the cherries. This is done by a machine which mashes the cherry and separates the beans. Then cleaning, washing and drying processes are usually carried out prior to roasting the coffee beans. Sometimes, to remove the outer coating or jelly-like layer around the beans, they are fermented for 12-18 hours in water; this is called controlled fermentation. After the beans are cleaned, they are sorted according to size. Then they are taken for roasting, where temperature and timing, colour and moisture levels are strictly controlled. Great care is taken over the roasting process to extract the full flavour from each bean. Once the process is completed, the beans are either sold as roasted coffee or go for grinding and then finally packing.

There are many varieties of coffee beans: some names are Bourbon, Typical, and Caturra. Each one has unique characteristics but the way the coffee is processed, shipped, stored, roasted, packaged and brewed all have a significant impact on taste.

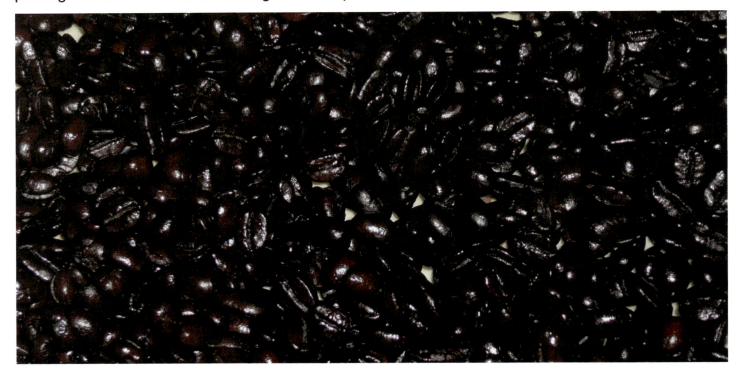

Roasted coffee beans

WHAT ARE THE HEALTH ISSUES?

Thermal stress during roasting, pesticide poisoning (plantation related), and allergic disorders affecting the eyes (conjunctivitis), skin or respiratory system are some of the health issues among workers in the coffee industry. The effects on respiratory systems are usually in the form of bronchitis or rhinitis and occupational asthma (Green coffee related). Repetitive strain and back-related muscular disorders, and noise-related hearing loss, have also been reported.

Chapter 7: Embriodery

Embroidery is the art of decorating existing fabrics or materials with needle and thread or yarn. It can be done by hand or machine. The fabrics (materials) are mostly woven textiles, but animal skins (goat, sheep, calf), bark, canvas are also used, and the decorative materials may include metal, glass, plastic, mirrors, beads, stone, ivory, feather, bone, horn, teeth, fish skin, beetle wing, tassels, buttons, coins, gemstones and coral.

The basic technology of embroidery is stitching. The threads or yarns used for stitching include cotton, silk, linen, wool, silver, gold and hair. Firstly designs are drawn on the fabrics and then threads are applied with a needle, or sometimes with a hook. There are generally three types of stitches and these are classified as *flat stitches*, *loop stitches* and *knotted stitches*. *Flat stitches* are so called because the threads lie flat on the surface of the fabrics; there are variations in flat stitches such as satin stitch, stem stitch, long and short stitch, cross stitch, tent stitch and couching. *Loop-forming stitches* are either open or closed. The open form is called buttonhole stitch and the closed one is called chain stitch. In *knotted stitches*, the knot is usually made on the fabric in the form of a French or Pekin knot.

In certain cultures, embroidery is a traditional craft, carried out by women from generation to generation. Some men and women practise this handicraft as a hobby, whereas in professional activities or in the embroidery industry, men, woman and children are all employed.

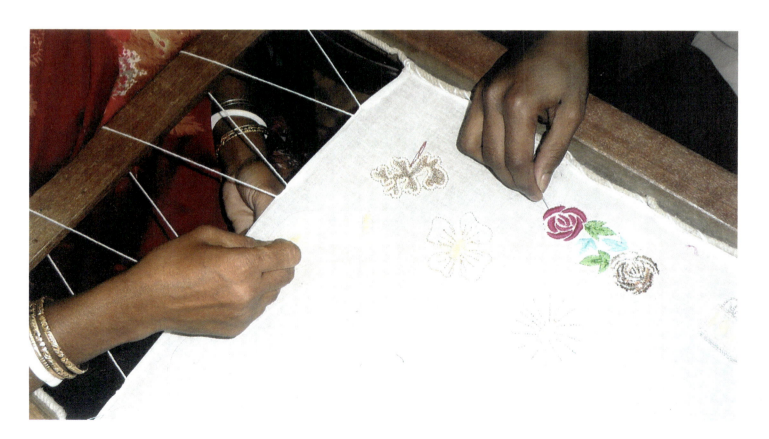

Woman and man engaged in embroidery work
(India)

18 Although ancient, the art of embroidery is practised throughout the world; regional characteristics are usually indentified by their presentation. Religion has a great impact on embroidery: all the major religions of the world, including Taoism, Hinduism, Buddhism, Christianity, Islam and Zoroastrianism, have influenced the patterns of embroidered textiles. Embroidered robes are used by many priests in various religious ceremonies. Births, marriages, burials, funerals and other special occasions or festivities are celebrated with embroidery. In certain countries embroidery has a great role in national costume or garments.

Embroidery is an ancient art and its precise time of discovery is very difficult to tell; examples were found in the tombs of Tuthmosis IV (resigned 1412-1364 BC) and Tutankhamun (resigned1334-1325 BC) in Egypt. An archaeological discovery in China indicates that silk embroidery has been practised in China since the third to fifth century BC.

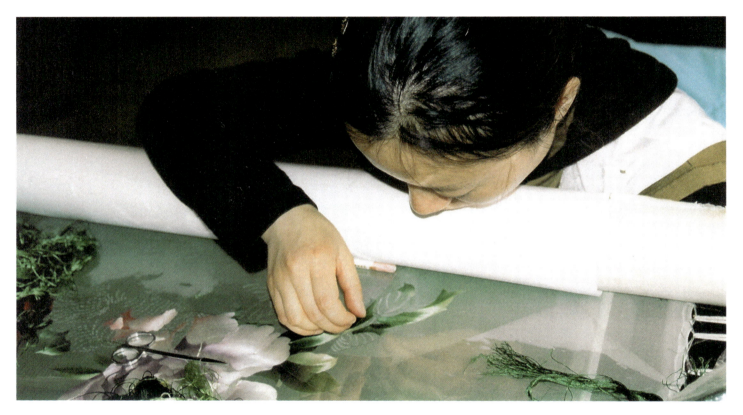

Chinese woman working on a silk embroidery (China)

The use of machines in embroidery started in the eighteenth century and nowadays a computerized embroidery machine is used for the pattern.

WHAT ARE THE HEALTH ISSUES?

Musculo-skeletal issues, eye symptoms, poor vision, dermatitis, friction burns and injuries, and work fatigue are the health-related issues affecting embroiderers. Sharp-tool-related injuries and posture-related back and upper limb disorders have been reported.

Chapter 8: Glass Making

Glass usually takes the form of hard, brittle, transparent and translucent objects whose uses we know: bottles, drinking glasses, glass jugs and jars, mirrors, eye wear (spectacles), windows, electric-light bulbs and so on.

The earliest glass known to have been used by man is natural glass. Lightning, heat and volcanic eruption sometimes fuse rocks and sands into a natural glass. Obsidian is one such kind of natural glass which was first used by ancient man as spearheads, arrowheads, knives and jewellery. Archaeological evidence suggests that man-made glass was first made in the form of a glaze about 6,000 years ago, although it is also sometimes said that glass was invented 4,500 years ago in Mesopotamia. In the fifteenth century BC the Egyptians were the first to produce glass from silica and potash. The technique of glass blowing was invented in the first century BC. In the fifteenth to nineteenth centuries Venice was supreme in glass making in Europe. The heyday of British glass-making was the seventeenth to nineteenth centuries. In the eighteenth century, semi-automatic processes were introduced instead of traditional mouth-blowing in glass-making technique; the first fully automated machine developed at the beginning of the nineteenth century.

Glass making at present is a modern hi-tech industry rather than just a traditional art or craft, and science plays a major role in its development. The materials used for making glass are sand, silica, soda ash (sodium oxide), lime (calcium oxide), and recycled glass (cullet). To make ordinary glass those are loaded at a high temperature into the glass-making furnaces.

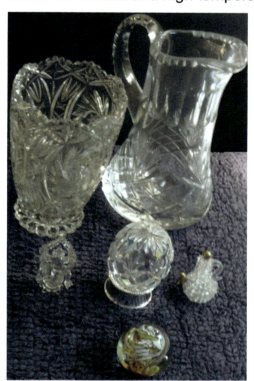

Ornamental glassware and Art objects

Thus the main components of glass making are i) silica, ii) alkaline flux (sodium and potassium) and iii) stabilizer (lime or lead oxide).

Coloured or opaque glass is made by adding compounds of metal oxides such as copper, chromium, nickel, cobalt, manganese and iron.

Lead glass (flint glass) contains a high proportion of lead oxide (red oxide): it is used for top-quality tableware and also for optical purposes. High-lead-content glass is used in the atomic energy industry, where the lead helps to guard against the harmful effects of radiation.

Crystal glass is made by melting a mixture of silica sand, borax, limestone, dolomite, potash and barium carbonate. Adding barium makes the brilliance of the crystal. To obtain this brilliance lead was once used, but has now been replaced by barium. Heat-resistant glass such as Pyrex (borosilicate glass) is made from silica and boric acid. It is used for cooking utensils, industrial pipes and laboratory equipment. Some glassware is microwavable. Corelle glass is one such product which is famous for durability, strength and lightness. It is usually made of three layers of glasses: core glass in the middle, with top and bottom layers of very thin or glaze glass.

Safety glass is a special types of glass which is usually tough and laminated; it is used in windscreens in the automobile industry and for windshields in aircraft. Modern flat glass windows are made by the float glass process. This type of flat sheet is made by floating molten glass on a bed of molten tin. Spectacle lenses, optical glass/fibres and optical instruments are another category of high purity glass. Fine fibres can be made from glass and these are known as fibreglass or glass wool; it is used as thermal insulator and in fabrics for curtains, tablecloths and construction.

20 Once the molten glass leaves the glass making furnace the shaping of the glass begins. The glassmaker gathers molten glass on the end of a hollow iron rod for blowing air.

Blowing is traditionally done with the mouth, so that a bubble is formed at the end of the hollow rod, which is then stretched and shaped with various hand-held tools – although nowadays in most places blowing is done by high speed automatic machines.

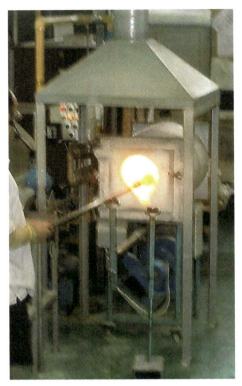

Glass-making furnace and molten glass

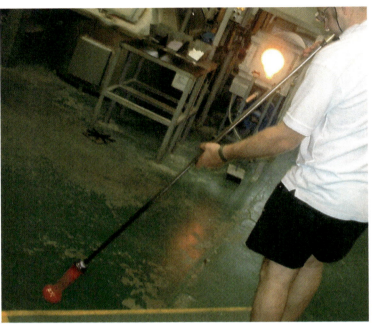

Glassmaker engaged in glass blowing

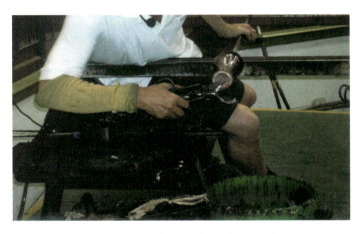

Shaping and cutting the glass

For shaping and making the various kinds of glasses there are also other methods such as pressing, casting and tubing.
However, whatever methods are used, once the glass is shaped, it undergoes annealing. Annealing is a process by which the glass is reheated followed by slow cooling; this is done to prevent stress fractures forming in the glass. Plain glassware is usually beautified by decorating it. This is usually done by cutting, grinding, engraving, etching, painting, sandblasting and/or colouring.

WHAT ARE THE HEALTH ISSUES?

Work-related accidents in the form of cuts, abrasions, lacerations, burns, fracture and eye injuries are not uncommon in the glass industry. Respiratory diseases like silicosis and tuberculosis have been reported. Heat stress, hearing loss, eye disorders, dermatitis and musculo-skeletal disorders are also found. Musculo-skeletal disorders and respiratory diseases have also been reported among child labourers in India. Some studies in Sweden, the USA, the UK and other countries in Europe have showed a slight risk of certain types of cancer (lung cancer, non-Hodgkin leukaemia) in the glass industry.

Chapter 9: Lace Making

Lace is an openwork fabric formed by removing threads or cloth from previously woven fabric, or patterned by looping, plaiting or twisting threads with a needle or set of bobbins. Lace work is mostly seen in garments and dress making (including wedding dresses), nets, curtains, pillow cases, covers, bed sheets, table cloths, cushions, and other items for internal decoration or for artistic work.

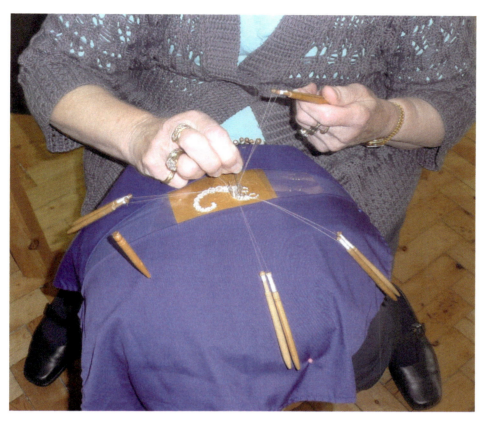

Honiton lace making at Allhallows Museum, Honiton, UK

Types of lace are classified on the basis of how they are constructed. For example, where needle and thread are used the result is *needle lace*; where lace is made with bobbins the result is called *bobbin lace*; where hook is used it is called *crochet lace*. *Filet lace* is netting, joined by knots. *Macramé* (an Arabic word) is a type of lace work made with knots and plaited threads. *Openwork* or *cutwork* is a kind of lace made by removing threads from linen cloth. *Embroidered lace* is open work on fabric or linen which is filled with embroidery. *Knitted lace* is a kind of knitting where holes are arranged or designed such a way as to give a natural or artistic beauty to the fabric. *Tape lace* is a type of lace where a pattern is made on a textile strip (tape) and then joined to the fabric. Sometimes the edge of a piece of cloth is lined or finished with lace and this type of lace trimming is called *hemming*. Lace which is not bleached is called *ecru lace*.

In England, Honiton is a town in Devon where famous *Honiton lace* is made and its existence is recorded since the early seventeenth century. The lace is made by hand and the bobbins are used for weaving process. The loom is being made from pins placed through a pattern on a straw pillow. The steps are to prepare the pattern, to wind the bobbins (twisting and braiding threads) and to make lace. The reef not is used to tie the knots between threads.

22 Scissors are used to cut the threads. To make a long piece of lace several laces are joined together.

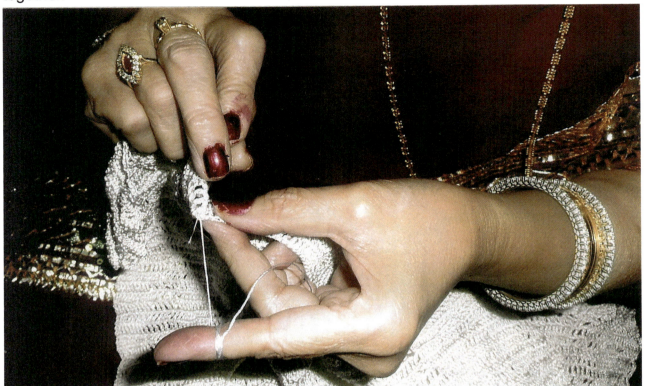

Crochet Lace knitting, India

Lace can be hand made or machine made. The lace-making machine was invented in the nineteenth century and since then machine-made lace has been produced, but demand for hand-made lace has not decreased. It is very difficult to determine when and where the first lace was made and who first invented lace making. Historically, this handicraft is an ancient art, as primitive peoples used it to make fishing nets for their livelihood. Modern lace making as an art and craft most probably began in Europe in the early fourteenth century on the border between France and present day Belgium; although lace-bobbin-like objects have been discovered in Roman ruins, there is no record to support Roman lace making. The clergy of the early Catholic Church might have used lace in religious ceremonial garments, but the popularity of lace making as a cottage industry began throughout Europe in the sixteenth century, and girls were employed. It spread to North America in the nineteenth century.

Lace-making materials are cotton, synthetic threads, silk, gold, silver and copper. The main tools are needles, bobbins and crochets, depending on the type of lace making. Bobbins are usually made of wood, bone or ivory. Scissors are also needed. Designing, tracing, ironing, washing, cleaning, colouring and bleaching are all part of the lace-making process. Materials used include linen, starch paste, resin, glue, chlorine and other bleaching or colouring agents.

WHAT ARE THE HEALTH ISSUES?

Needle puncture injuries, twisting injuries, repetitive strain injuries, musculo-skeletal disorders, eye strain, dust and skin disorders can occur amongst lace makers. Posture-related musculo-skeletal disorders involving the neck, shoulder and back have been reported amongst hand-made lace makers.Some of the chemicals used during lace-making processes are known respiratory irritants, skin sensitizers, or carcinogenic agents.

Chapter 10: Lavender

Lavender is a flowering plant from which various toiletries, oils and household products are made. The plant is well known as a fragrant herb and there are 39 varieties. A lavender plant consists of stem, spike, leaves and flowers; the stalks are tied in bundles when the stems are cut. The colour of the leaves and flowers depends on the type species. The leaves can be green, grey, dark green or yellow green. Flowers can be blue, violet, purple, pink, lemon chiffon or lilac. The name 'lavender', which was given by the Romans, comes from the Latin word *lavare* meaning 'to wash'. The Greeks referred to it as 'nardus' after the city of Naardus in Syria. The people of India called it 'spikenard'; the name originated from the shape of the flower. The ancient Egyptians used lavender for mummification as well as perfumes. Romans used lavender oil in bathing and cooking, as a scent and disinfectant, and for washing clothes. Originally the plant grew in the Mediterranean region (southern Europe, North Africa), Asia Minor and India; it now grows all over the world. The Provence region of France is the world's largest lavender-producing region and this lavender is widely used in the perfume industry. Commercially lavender is also grown in Spain, Italy, England, Bulgaria, the USA, Australia, South Africa, New Zealand and Japan.

Its commercial uses include cosmetics, medicinal products, crafts, potpourri, bouquets, candles and culinary purposes. Lavender has therapeutic, antimicrobial properties and is also used in aromatherapy.

Lavender production varies from country to country, place to place and region to region, as growth depends on climate, soil conditions, type of lavender and harvesting. French lavender is *lavendula dentata*, which is a tender lavender that grows in southern France and Spain in full sun, whereas English lavender is *lavendula angustifolia*, a hardy lavender that grows in the long daylight of the English summer (April to July). The heat of the sun may not be as strong as in France or Spain, but the plant needs at least six hours of direct sun on average each day. The soil is usually alkaline. Pruning is done in August. In lavender cultivation pesticides and herbicides are usually avoided. Lavender fields rarely need fertilizer, but compost is used to balance the Ph. Soil solarisation is needed and watering may be required to counteract dryness. In India lavender grows in the Himalaya region and the variety is *Lavendula officinalis*, which is sweet lavender. There are four varieties of English lavender: Folgate, Imperial Gem, Maillette and Grosso.

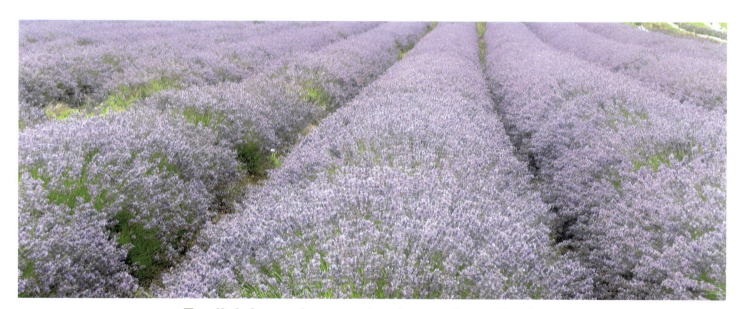

English lavender growing in southern England

24 Lavender is usually distilled to produce essential oil by the process of steam distillation.

To make essential oil from lavender, certain processes are involved. After harvesting, the spikes of lavender are cut and dried. The dried lavender is put in the tank of the still (the apparatus for distillation) and water is added. The still is packed tightly by adding further raw material (lavender plants). The still is then closed and the water is heated to between 100° and 212°C. The distillate starts to come out through the condenser and into the separator. Once the distillation is complete, the collected oil is filtered.

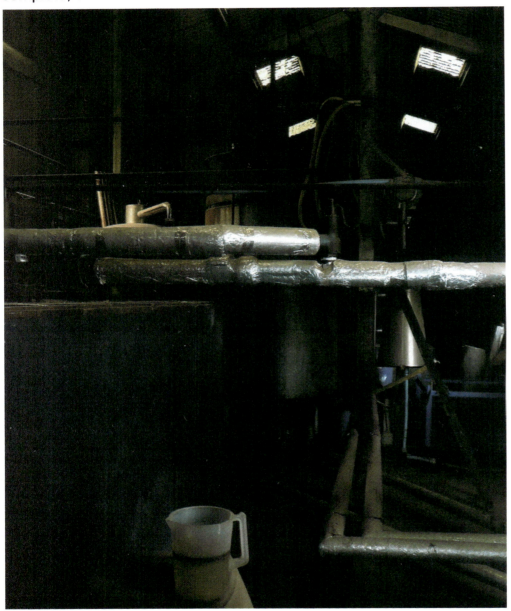

Distillation process for lavender

The distillation process produces the essential oil and hydrosol.
The hydrosol can be reused or discarded.
In the process the apparatuses involved are:

a) furnace, for heating by direct fire, gas or electricity

b) holding tank, for adding water and raw materials

c) condenser, for collecting and cooling the raised steam after heating

d) separator, for separating essential oils from water vapour.

WHAT ARE THE HEALTH ISSUES?

Lavender cultivation does not involve any pesticides or herbicides or fertilizer-related chemical hazards. However, hydrosol- or distillation-water-related health hazards (bacterial and fungal infections) cannot be ruled out, as bacteria and fungi can easily grow in hydrosol. Lavender-related fire hazards have also been reported as lavender is highly inflammable.

Chapter 11: Leather

British Standard BS 2780 defines leather as hide or skin with its original fibrous structure more or less intact, tanned to be imputrescible. The hair or wool may or may not have been removed. It can also be made from a hide or skin that has been split into layers or segmented either before or after tanning.

Primitive man used raw hide and stone tools prior to 40,000 BC for scraping animal skins. Flint tools were being used for puncturing holes in the skin prior to 10,000 BC. Around 10,000 BC, bone tools were used for scraping hides and skins to remove hair. Shoes dating from the Bronze Age have been found in the Alps, made from bear and deer skin. In ancient Egypt, leather was used for sandals, clothes, gloves, buckets, bottles, shrouds for burying the dead and for military equipment: all of these have been discovered among the paintings and artefacts in excavated tombs.In ancient India, the sadhus and rishis used mats which were prepared from the skins of animals like tigers and deer. Also in ancient India, the leather processing trade was run by a particular caste, the *Mochi*. *Mochis* are still found in the streets of India and they mostly work as cobblers.

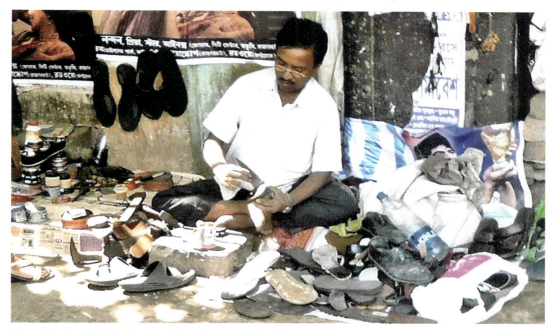

Mochi (cobbler) on the footpath, busy with shoe repair work (India)

The trade of leather tanning was developed in India by around 3,000 BC. The Greek and Roman civilisations also gave the greatest importance to the tanning of leather. The uses of leather in ancient Greece and in the Roman Empire were widespread. In the Roman Empire leather was commonly used in the form of footwear, clothes, and military equipment, including shields, saddles and harnesses. It was the Romans who brought the art of leather making to Britain. From the late nineteenth century onwards, with the general rise in living standards, the demand for leather products has increased throughout the world. The major leather-producing countries are Argentina, Australia, Brazil, China, Italy, India, the USA and the USSR, although developing countries now produce over 60% of the world's leather. Leather products include footwear, bags, wallets, straps, belts, watchstraps, seats, armrests, harnesses, luggage, clothing, caps, saddles, bullwhips, water carriers and other goods. They are made from the hides of cattle, lambs, goats, sheep, pigs, deer, buffalo, dogs, snakes, alligators, ostriches, kangaroos, oxen, yaks, stingrays and various other animals, although most leather products from some animal skins are banned due to animal conservation issues.

26   The leather manufacturing process consists of four stages:

    a)   The first is the 'preparatory stage', when the hide is prepared for tanning. The steps are preservation (curing), soaking, painting, liming, fleshing, de-liming, bating, pickling and degreasing.

b)   The second stage is 'tanning'. Most leather is tanned using salts of chromium. Other substances are aldehyde, oils and vegetable tanning. Vegetable tanning agents are various plant extracts, such as saffron, indigo, oak, chestnut and hemlock.

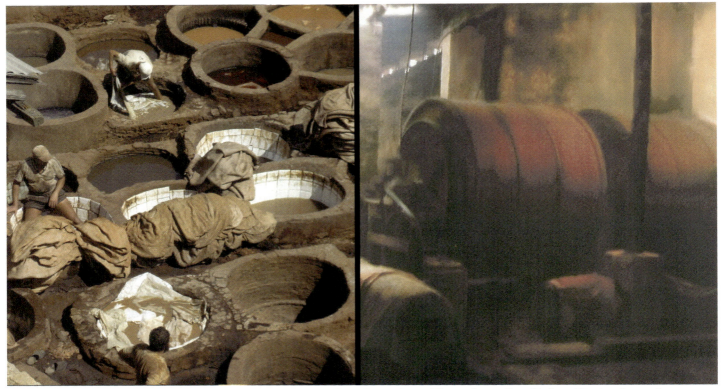

Traditional Leather Tanning (Morocco)   Leather Tanning (India) - Rotating drums

c)   The third stage is the 'crusting operation', which involves shamming, splitting, shaving, neutralisation, dyeing, fat liquoring, setting, drying, staking and buffing.

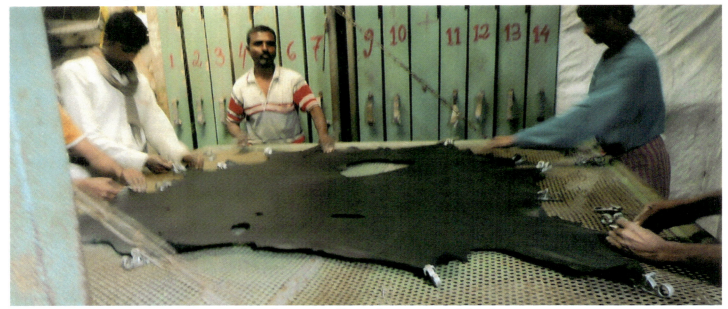

Setting out (Leather stretching)

d) The final stage is 'finishing'. The objects of this process are i) to level the colour, ii) to cover the defects, iii) to control the gloss and iv) to provide a protective surface. The operation may include oiling, brushing, padding, spraying, coating, polishing, plating and ironing.

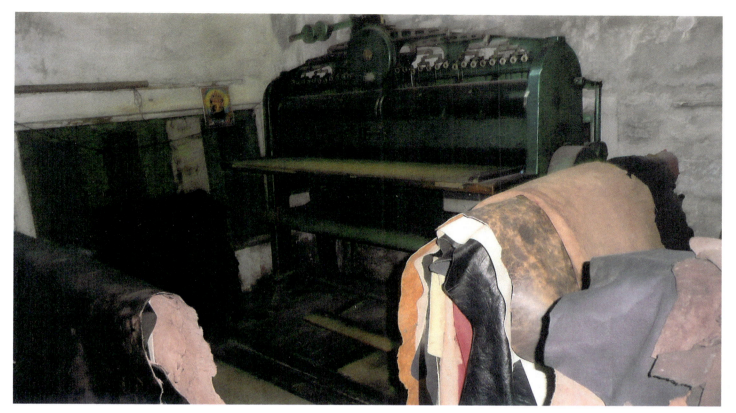

Finished leather before despatch

Before despatch to the customer, the finished leather is graded and each piece is measured.

WHAT ARE THE HEALTH ISSUES?

They include:
a)   Injuries due to slips, falls, burns and cuts.
b)   Noise-related deafness.
c)   Infections such as anthrax and brucellosis from raw hides and skins
d)   Dermatitis, allergies and ulceration of the skin, including perforation of the nasal septum by chromium salts.
e)   Dust- and chemical-induced chronic bronchitis.
f)   Increased incidence of cancer of the nasal passages due to leather dust. Other probable leather-related cancer hazards are, i) lung cancer, ii) pancreatic cancer, iii) bladder cancer, iv) testicular cancer, and v) leukaemia.
g)   Peripheral neuropathy (shoemaker neuropathy) has been reported in some European countries due to inhalation of solvents (N-hexane) in the leather adhesive.
h)   Waste discharges which pollute air, water and soil can cause asthma, dermatitis, hepatic, neurological and malignancy disorders.

Chapter 12: Mask Making

A mask is a face covering, usually worn to protect or disguise the face.

Mask making is an art whose history goes back to 20,000 BC. Although it is not exactly known when or why people started to create masks, it is certain that hunters and gatherers created masks from natural products (animal skins, animal bones, branches, grasses, leaves, feathers etc.) to try to sneak up on animals.

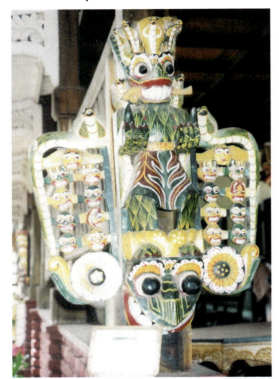

Maha Kola (Devil dance Mask- commands 18 demons of illness), Sri Lanka

Since ancient times and throughout human civilisation masks have had a significant role, particularly warrior masks, armour, masks used in healing activities (physician's mask), death masks and other religious rituals.

The Greeks and Romans introduced masks in theatrical productions. Masks are now used in costume parties, carnivals, festivals, and by performers such as dancers, comedians and actors. Children also love to dress up.

Civilisations which are or were traditionally users of masks are the Egyptian, Chinese, Greek and Roman; countries where they are used include Italy, many parts of Africa, India, Japan, Australia, Sri Lanka, Thailand, Mexico and America. Each country has its own style of making masks, but the basic principles are more or less the same everywhere.

Protective masks are mainly safety or occupational masks, such as welders' masks, gas masks and radiation protection workers' mask, or devices to protect against other health hazards. There are also radiotherapy masks, worn during radiotherapy investigation and treatment.

Masks are also used in medical and cosmetic procedures, as disguises, in sports (hockey, fencing) and in the fashion industry.

There are many ways of making masks and the techniques of mask making include sculpting, moulding, casting, fabricating, decorating and painting. The procedure also depends on the types of materials available in particular places, the types of materials individuals choose and the methods used. However, it largely involves work with clay, wood, plaster, cement, plastic, acrylic, metals, latex, neoprene, vinyl, PVC, foam, papier maché, leather, silicone, paint, fur, feathers, hair, teeth, horn, sea shells, glass, porcelain and so on. The tools used also depend on the types of materials one is working on.

For example, for a *leather mask*, the tools are usually a sharp knife or scalpel, fabric shears, steel straight edge and modelling spatula. Leather mask making begins with softening the leather. This is done by placing the leather in warm water and then draining and leaving it to dry at least for thirty minutes. To make a mould shape, the leather is bent, stretched and creased. To colour it, dyes or paints are used. For that, brushes, applicators or sponges are required. A cloth is used to dry and burnish; then necessary decorations are added and the mask is finished by applying metallic finish or by glazing or varnishing.

For a *wooden mask*, the tools needed are wood saw, drill, chisels, wood carving knives, wood glue and decorating materials such as paints, features, glitter etc.

The method is to make a sketch on paper and then cut the wood to the right size and shape on the basis of the sketch. Drill the holes for an eye, mouth, and nose and carve the wood to the desired design, making further holes if necessary. Paint the wood or attach the feathers, glitter or other decorating materials.

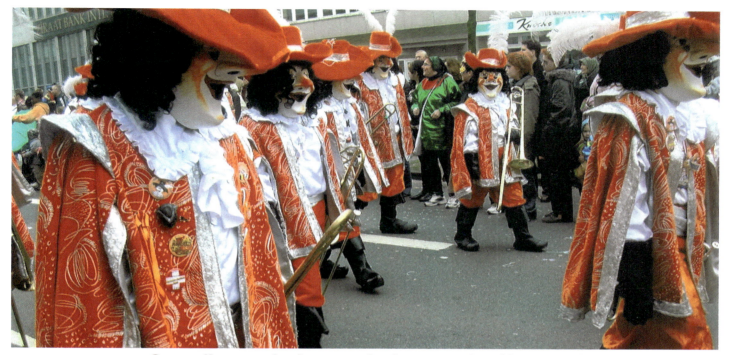

Comedian masks in a carnival procession (Germany)

For a *papier maché mask*, the materials are: a) aluminium foil or a balloon or cardboard or chicken wire (used as base or form), b) newspaper, c) papier maché paste (a thick glue made by mixing flour and water), d) hole punch, e) elastic cord, f) paint. The steps are:

Step one - Prepare the desired quantity of papier maché paste.

Step two - Tear the newspapers into strips.

Step three- Dip one piece of newspaper at a time into prepared maché paste.

Step four - Stick the newspaper strips over the base or on the form. After one layer is applied, let it dry completely. Add a second layer of newspaper strips and let it dry completely. Continue this process until the desired effect is achieved.

Step five- Cover one side of the base or form, making sure there are holes for eyes; add features like a nose, ears, and eyebrows and then apply final layer of papier maché strips and let it dry.

Step six- Make a hole in each side of the mask, using a hole punch; run a piece of elastic cord through the holes and tie in a knot at each end.

Step seven:- Finally, paint or decorate as desired.

To make a *plaster mask*, a human volunteer is needed for casting. Apply Vaseline and then use plaster of paris gauze bandage strips (a 3-inch roll) to the face of the volunteer. This is usually done by dunking the plaster bandage in a bowl of water at room temperature, squeezing out excess water and then applying the strips to the face, so that the covering is gradually widened and thickened. Certain areas of the face need building up: this is usually done by reinforcing the bandages on the nose, cheeks etc. The built-up mask is taken off once the volunteer feels that the mask is pulling away from his face. Once the plaster cast mask is removed, if necessary put more plaster gauze on areas that are found to be too light. Let it dry completely, then finish it by applying the desired painting and decorating.

30 To make a *clay mask*, the clay is firstly cut from a block of clay and then rolled out using a slab roller. A mould is needed to create a pottery mask. Sculpting of the face is done from the mould, taken from the clay. Facial features are made by pushing, pressing, punching and trimming. For this, needle tools and trimming tools are needed. A ceramic mask is glazed and painted before it goes for firing.

For *plastic mask* making, a face mould made of plaster of paris or wood is required. A thin white acrylic or PVC sheet is necessary which is usually softened in an oven. Once it is softened, the cut-out sheet is taken from the oven, pushed down over the mould and held in place as it cools. It is then lubricated and a negative cast made in the plaster of Paris. Then a plastic sheet is laid down over the mould so a postive mask can be made. The positive and negative formers can then be used in a press for mask production.

A *neoprene mask* can be made by casting the mask with neoprene rubber which requires appropriate trimming and sanding.

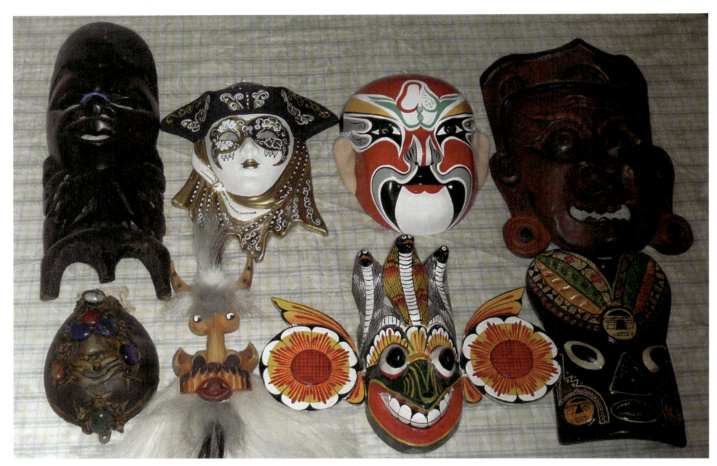

Masks from Africa, Italy, China, India, Bolivia, Bulgaria, Sri Lanka and Peru (Author's collection)

WHAT ARE THE HEALTH ISSUES?

Tool-related injuries, including knife cuts, during mask-making processes have been reported. Health issues depend on the types of materials in use during handling as well as due to process related exposure; the affects are mostly musculo-skeletal, skin-related (dermatitis) or respiratory (occupational asthma or irritation).

Paper making is the process of making paper, which is a kind of material mainly used for writing, printing, and packaging and in cleaning products. It is produced from connected fibres such as cellulose (from plants, including trees), cotton and linen fibres or cloth rags.

The word paper is derived from the Greek term for 'papyrus', which was used for writing on by the ancient Egyptians. This was formed from beaten strips of the papyrus plant.

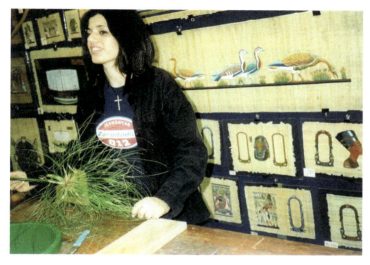

Paper making from the papyrus plant in Egypt

Modern paper making is said to have been invented in China in about 100 AD. The first pulp-paper-making process was developed in China during the early second century AD and from China it spread to the Islamic world. The Chinese and Muslims used human- and animal-powered mills in the paper-making process. However, the first water-powered paper mill was built in Europe in the thirteenth century. In 1884, the process for pulping wood for paper-making began. The main categories of paper products are currently writing and printing papers, newsprint and magazine papers, sanitary and household, packaging materials and specialised papers like currency etc. The top ten paper-making countries of the world are the USA, Japan, China, Canada, Germany, Finland, Sweden, France, Korea and Italy.

In the paper-making process the raw materials are wood-based forest products from trees. There are two types: one is softwood from coniferous trees (spruce and fir) to make stronger paper; the other is hardwood from deciduous trees (leafy trees such as poplar and elm). Other than trees, paper makers also use plant fibres such as bamboo, straw, sugar cane, flex, hemp and jute. Other types of fibres are wood fibres from sawmills, vegetable fibres, recycled papers and cloths. Many countries now uses up to 40% recycled paper during the paper-making process: the paper is shredded and mixed with water. Cloths are cotton and linen rags. Rags are usually cuttings and waste from textile and garment mills. Rags must be cut, boiled and beaten before they can be used by the paper mill.

Most papers are made from wood pulp. The wood is converted into pulp either mechanically or chemically. In the mechanical method, the logs are first tumbled in drums to remove the bark and then fed into a set of revolving grindstones. The grinders break the wood down to a pulp: thus the wood leaves the grinder as a fine, wet pulpy mass. The pulp is then filtered to remove foreign objects.

In the chemical process, the debarked logs are cut into small pieces (wood chips) and the wood chips are cooked in a chemical solution in a sealed vessel (digester). Sulphites are used in acid processing and sulphates in alkaline processing. The chemical action takes place and dissolves substances like lignin, which binds the cellulose fibres together. Next the pulp is sent through filters before it goes to the paper-making plant for further processing.

In the paper-making plant, the pulp is beaten by beaters and then mixed with other substances such as:

i)   bleaches (chlorine and hypochlorite), dyes and pigments,
ii) fillers (chalk, clay, titanium oxide),
iii) sizings (rosin, alum, gum, starch) in a mixer to produce the types of paper desired.

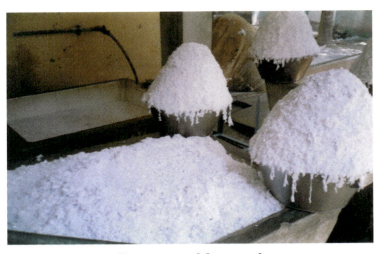

Paper making pulp

It then flows into a machine which drains off the water, after which the damp paper is dried into a continuous sheet. It is then passed through a wire-mesh belt, where most of the remaining water drains or is sucked away. The damp web of paper leaving the wire-mesh belt is led through a succession of drying cylinders and press rollers. The dried paper is then wound onto large reels, and will be further processed depending on its ultimate use.

The finishing process involves:
a)   smoothing,
b)   making the surface soft and dull or hard and shiny by passing through metal rollers (calendars),
c)   coating by adding chemicals or pigments.
Finally, the paper is cut to the desired size.

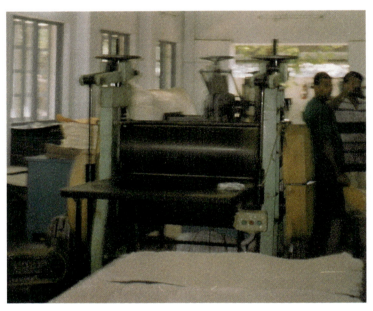

Rollers for the finishing process

WHAT ARE THE HEALTH ISSUES?

Air and water pollution is the most important issue in the pulp and paper industry. Chemicals like dioxins, furans and other organochlorines are discharged from pulp and paper mills into surface water. The chemical-related health hazards are headache, nausea, eye and breathing irritation, and dermatitis. People who suffer from asthma, emphysema or chronic obstructive airways diseases (COPD) may find that their episodes increase. The physical hazards include accidents, injuries, noise and musculo-skeletal disorders. Increased risk of lung cancer, malignant lymphoma and stomach cancer has been reported amongst workers in the pulp and paper industry.

Most plastics are chemically produced substances whose characteristics of plasticity or malleability make them easily moulded or shaped. Plastic materials have now significantly replaced traditional wood, glass and textile materials in domestic, commercial and industrial uses. Toys, dolls, kitchen utensils, bottles, switches, clothing, bags, carpets and so on are the prime examples of plastic in use. Some plastics are natural and some are synthetic.

In the eighteenth century, the first man-made plastic was invented and its development was a gradual process. It started with the use of natural plastic materials, then chemically modified natural materials and finally the full synthetic materials were invented. Natural plastics are made from plants and insects such as latex from rubber trees, rosin from pine trees and shellac from lac insects. The chemically modified natural plastics are synthetic rubber, nitrocellulose, collagen and galalite. Acrylics, amino resins, epoxy resins, polyurethane and vinyl chlorides are the synthetic plastics, which are made from chemicals such as crude oil, petroleum and coal. They are usually manufactured by the process of polymerization. Thermoplastics and thermosetting are the two kinds of plastic: the difference depends on the procedures which are used to shape the plastics. Thermoplastics are types of plastics which melt easily if heated. Most of the common plastics are in this group. On the other hand, the chemical structure of thermosetting plastics is such that the plastic remains rigid when heated. Plastics are shaped in various ways by the process of moulding, extraction, calendaring, laminating and welding.

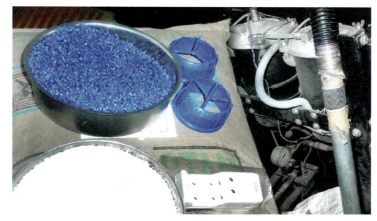

Plastic granules, the process and the finished products

The forms of some of the plastics are:
Nylon is a synthetic textile which is a fibrous form of plastic. It is formed either by the condensation of acid (adipic acid) and an amine (hexamethylenediamine) or by the polymerization of a lactam (caprolactam). Nylon plastics are moulded into various consumer products including house-wares and electrical appliances.

Acrylics are the polymerized esters such as methyl methacrylate, methyl acrylate, ethyl acrylate and butyl acrylate and the most common uses are as Perspex, Lucite, and Plexiglas, which are glass-like plastics, i.e. substitutes for glass.

They are also used in dentures, surgical prostheses, fibres and coatings for textiles, paper and leather as adhesives.

Amino resins are produced from a combination of formaldehyde and urea or melamine. They are used as resins and adhesives for plywood, foam insulation and particle board, and also for laminated objects, moulding compounds, surface coatings, paper coatings and textile printing.

Epoxy resins are formed by the reaction of two chemicals: one is a resin (epoxide) and other is a hardener (polyamine). Epoxy resins are used as adhesives, reinforcing agents, laminating materials, paints and surface coatings. They have great applications in the aerospace industry, in automobile, bicycle and boat making, and in the manufacturing of rotor blades for wind turbines. Epoxy resins are excellent electrical insulators that have important uses in the electrical and electronics industries.

Vinyl chloride is an organic chemical compound which is used to make PVC (poly vinyl chloride). PVC is very useful plastic which has wide uses. It is used to make pipes, electrical goods, cables, automobile parts, packing materials, household goods, shower curtains, window frames, flooring, raincoats, handbags, dresses, tape recorders, toy figurines and so on.

Polyurethane is a polymer. Polyurethane polymers are formed through the reaction of isocyanates (toluene diisocyanate, methylenediphenyl diisocyanate, hexamethylene diisocyanate) with di- or polyfunctional alcohols. This plastic has wide uses because of its stiffness, hardness and density. Polyurethane foams are used as cushioning foams, thermal insulation foams and packaging. Isocyanates are used in the production of adhesives, rubbers, printing rollers, surface coatings and spray paints.

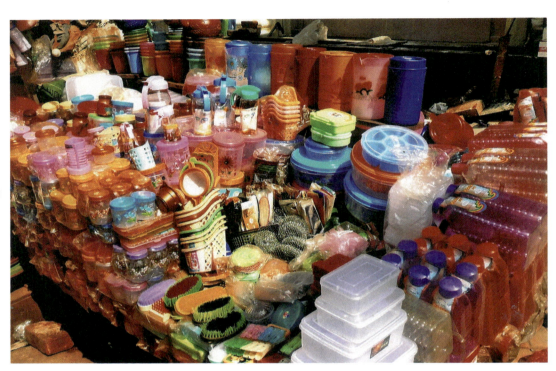

Plastic goods displayed at a roadside market in India

WHAT ARE THE HEALTH ISSUES?

Injuries can occur during manual handling, or from slipping or tripping; they may be machinery related or involve a blow from an object, including knife-cuts. Noise-related ill health, occupational asthma, respiratory irritation and dermatitis are the main concerns. However, more specific chemical-related diseases caused by various plastic manufacturing process are:

Nylon: adipic acid and caprolactin irritate the eyes, skin and throat. Asthma (adipic acid related) and bladder cancer mortality has been reported amongst nylon manufacturing workers.

Acrylics: manufacturing chemicals may cause dermatitis, asthma and peripheral neuropathy.

Amino resins: formaldehyde can cause dermatitis, asthma and in severe cases chemical pneumonitis or pulmonary oedema. Leukaemia has also been reported.

Epoxy resins: Epichlororohydrin, bisphenol A can cause asthma, rhinitis and dermatitis. There may be some risk of cancer of the lungs and pancreas and of reproductive toxin effects.

Vinyl chloride: has a toxic effect on the nervous system (headache, light-headedness, dizziness); it may affect the vascular and skeletal systems (Raynuad's phenomenon, scleroderma-like skin lesions, acro-osteolysis) or the hepatic system (hepatitis, cirrhosis) or respiratory system (asthma, pneumonitis, pulmonary fibrosis), There is also a risk of cancer affecting the liver, brain or blood (leukaemia).

Polyurethane: isocyanates can cause occupational asthma, chronic obstructive airways disease and pneumonitis. There may be a risk of non-Hodgkin's lymphoma, or rectal or pancreatic cancer.

Chapter 15: Pottery Making

Pottery is the craft of making pots from certain kinds of clay, especially by hand. Pottery-making clay usually contains silicate materials and kaolinite is the most important clay. The earliest pottery was made by hand and fired in bonfires. The uses of pottery were well known in ancient Egypt and in the Indus Valley and Sumerian civilisations. The earliest ceramic object discovered in Europe, in the Czech Republic, is a nude female figure dated to 29,000-25,000 BC. The earliest known pottery vessels made in Japan go back to around 10,500 BC. Pottery dating back to 10,000 BC has been excavated in China.

The invention of potter's wheel took place most probably in the mid-fourth millennium BC at Mesopotamia and the potter's kick wheel driven by the foot was invented in the first century. China is one of the countries where colouring of pottery first appeared: the ancient Chinese made blue coloured porcelain by using iron and red coloured from copper. However, over the years many additional tools and various machines have been gradually developed to manufacture pottery.

Earthenware, *stoneware* and *porcelain* are the main types of pottery.

Earthenware is the commonest, cheapest pottery and the easiest to make, using flint clay, bail clay or kaolin (china clay) and china stones. It is glazed and fired at a low temperature (about 1000°C to 1100°C).White glazed cups and plates which are in daily use are usually made of earthenware.

Stoneware is a very hard and strong kind of pottery. It is made from fire clay, ball clay, feldspar and silica and usually fired at a higher temperature (about 1200°C to 1300°C) than earthenware. Jugs, heavy dishes and jars are usually made of stoneware.

Porcelain is usually referred as china or chinaware because China is the birthplace of porcelain making. It is usually made from kaolin (china clay) and china stone and fired at the highest temperature (about 1400°C). Porcelain is famous for strength, toughness, whiteness, translucence and resistance to chemical change and thermal shock. Porcelain is used not only for making beautiful china but also as an excellent insulator in the electrical industry.

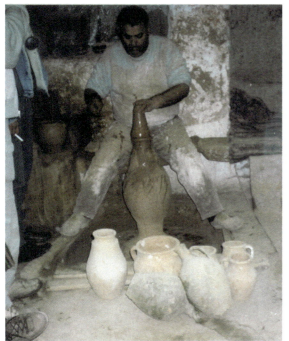

Shaping the pottery using a potter's kick wheel in Turkey

It is also used for table, kitchen and sanitary ware, tiles, and decorative and artistic objects. Porcelain made from paste and fired at a very high temperature is called hard-paste porcelain. Soft-paste porcelain is made from a mixture of white clay and a powdered mass of glass, sand or broken china and is fired at a lower temperature (less than 1100°C) than hard-paste porcelain.

Bone china is a kind of porcelain where bone ash (50%) is used as a main ingredient and rest is kaolin (china clay) and china stone. It is fired at 1240°C.

To manufacture pottery, the process involves shaping, firing, glazing and decorating. For shaping the pottery, the potter uses a potter's wheel, which is a device for rotating clay while the potter shapes it with his hands. The action of shaping the wet clay on the wheel is called *throwing*. During the process of *throwing*, the soft clay ball is pressed downwards and outwards symmetrically – this is called *centering* the clay – and the next step is *opening*, which means to make a hollow in the centre of the clay ball. Then *flooring* is done by making a flat and round-shaped bottom, after which the sides are shaped by

throwing or pulling. *Trimming* or *turning* is done by removing excess clay and refining the shape of the pot.

36 The method of hand *throwing* is gradually being replaced by a mechanical *throwing* process. *Jiggering* and *jolleying* operations take place by machine. *Jiggering* is used to make flat ware such as plates and jolleying is used for making hollow ware such as cups. Firing takes place in kilns. The kiln is usually heated by wood, coal, gas or electricity. Burning fuels may cause smoke, soot and ash.

A *glaze* is a glassy coating applied to pottery: this is done by dipping or pouring or by simply coating with a thin layer of a basic clay-like mixture, or making colours by adding certain metal oxides as ingredients. Salt, sulphur, tin, zinc, iron and copper salts are the various compounds which are used as glazing materials. Fluxes are lead, boron, potassium and sodium. Decorating pottery means patterning and/or painting the pottery; it can be done by incising patterns on the clay body, as on-glaze, in-glaze or under-glaze decoration, or by enamelling.

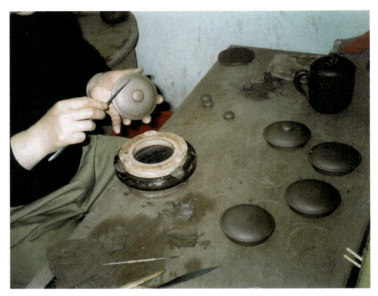
Triming and refining the earthenware

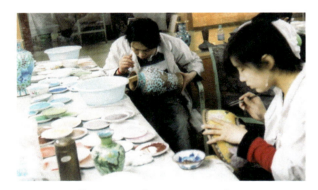
Decorating ceramics

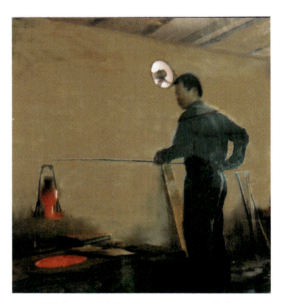
Firing Chinese porcelain

Jingdezhen in China is the only city in the world where the highest quantities of porcelain are made. Staffordshire in England is well known for bone china and the famous names in English pottery are Wedgewood and Dalton. Avanos in the Cappadocia region is the traditional pottery-making centre of Turkey, where the distinctive red clay from the river is used.

WHAT ARE THE HEALTH ISSUES?

These include injuries and burns while handling, lifting or carrying; slipping, tripping, falling or being hit by moving, flying or falling objects. The dust in the pottery industry contains large amounts of silica and silicosis is a frequently occurring disease. Other reported diseases are dermatitis, musculo-skeletal disorders such as carpal tunnel syndrome, traumatic tendonitis, RSI (repetitive strain injury) and occupational asthma. Besides, there may be some risk of lung and stomach cancer.

Chapter 16: Rope Making (Non-Metallic)

A rope is a stout cord, made of a bundle of flexible fibres which are twisted or braided to increase its overall length as well as tensile strength, so that it becomes strong, thick and flexible. Thanks to these properties it is used for connecting and pulling and thus the main users are fishing and maritime industries. Although the history of rope making from plant fibres (vines) goes back to prehistoric times, it was probably the ancient Egyptians who invented tools for making rope. About 5,500–6,000 years ago, they used materials like reeds, palms, papyrus, flex, grass, leather and animal furs to make ropes. Such ropes were used to pull and move the stones to build the pyramids. This art then most probably spread to Asia and Europe.

Since ancient times ropes have been used for hunting, carrying, lifting, pulling, attaching, fastening and climbing. In modern times their importance has spread to various fields such as construction, communication, exploration, seafaring and sports.

The sources of non-metallic rope fibres may be natural, synthetic or animal products. Natural fibres are mostly plant fibres such as cotton, linen, jute, coir, hemp and sisal. Synthetic fibres are nylon, polyesters, polypropylene, polyethylene, twaron, triptolon and rayon. Animal fibres include silk, wool and hair, but their use in rope for commercial purposes is rare. Sometimes rope is made by mixing several kinds of fibres. Rope making from coir fibres is quite popular as a cottage industry, especially in some of the coconut-growing regions of the world. India (Kerala) and Sri Lanka are the major coir-rope-making countries and India is the country where the craft is generally thought to have originated. Other countries like Mexico, Indonesia, Vietnam and the Caribbean islands also produce some coir. Coir fibres are found in between the husk and the outer shell of a coconut.

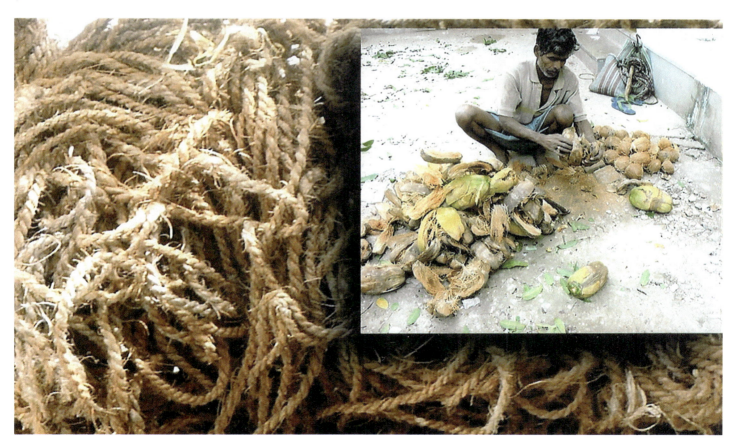

Rope from coir fibres

38 There are two types of fibres: one is brown fibre and the other is white fibre. It is mostly white fibres which are used for rope making. The immature husks are suspended in a water-filled pit or in a river for 9-10 months, during which the process of ratting (breakdown of the plant tissues by micro-organisms) takes place. The long fibres are separated by beating by hand and are then dried and cleaned. The cleaned fibres then go for spinning into yarn from which rope is manufactured. Nowadays machinery is also available to replace hand beating.

White jute (*corchorus capsularis*) fibres are also used to make the rope. Bangladesh, India (West Bengal) and China are the main countries where white jute is produced.

Nowadays synthetic fibres are popular for rope manufacturing and are no doubt replacing some of the plant fibres. Hemp, sisal and cotton are being replaced by plastic materials because of the worldwide demand for stronger ropes. Polypropylene is widely used for ropes because it is light enough to float. Twaron and triptolon (respectively an aramid and a polyaramid) are used because of their heat-resistant properties. Nylon has an elastic stretch property. Polyester is a strong, abrasion-resistant and stretches less under load. Braided ropes are usually made from these synthetic fibres.

Rope can be manufactured in three ways: one is called twisted rope and the other two are braided rope and plaited rope. All three involve making yarn by twisting fibres together. For twisted ropes, the yarn is twisted into stands and then the strands are twisted into rope. For braided rope, the yarn is braided rather than being twisted into strands. Plaited rope is made by braiding twisted strands. A rope walk is a space, over 400 yards long, where actual making or laying of ropes takes place. Colouring or coloured ropes are made by dyeing the rope or rope fibres.

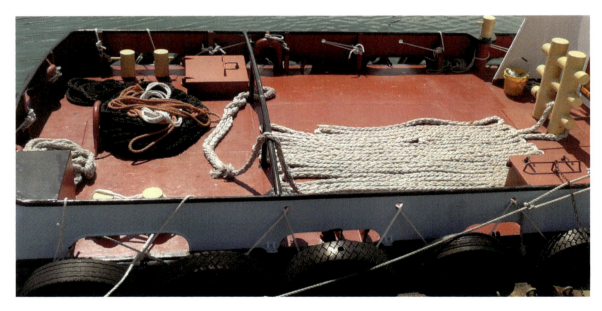

Tugboat rope (Bedded and twisted synthetic fibres)

WHAT ARE THE HEALTH ISSUES?

Accidental injuries, including musculo-skeletal injuries as a result of manual handling, or from slips, trips or falls or from moving machinery, can occur. Friction burns from handling fibres or cord are not uncommon. Noise-induced deafness has been reported. During braiding work, the braider makes lots of dexterity movements in the form of flexions, extensions, pronations and supernations, which can give rise to tenosinovitis or peritendinitis crepitus.

Some rope fibres can cause eye, skin and respiratory tract irritation. They may be responsible for dust-related respiratory disorders. Skin disorders like dermatitis, oil folliculitis and hyperkeratosis can occur. Some synthetic plastic fibres such as nylon, polyester, and polypropylene may increased the risk of certain cancers (bladder,colon).

It is very difficult to say whether or not the ancient world gave any important to rubber cultivation, but the modern world certainly does because of the commercial benefits. However, the waterproofing and elastic properties of various rubber-producing plants were discovered by native Americans, the Aztecs or earlier Mesoamericans and South American tribes. The ancient tribes must have used the rubber to make various artefacts and ornaments, and utilised its adhesive properties for making arrows and bows. In the rainforests of Ecuador, the local natives used natural rubber for waterproof boots, bottles etc.

Natural rubber is the solid elastic material which is isolated after wounding the plant, and it is mostly a white milky fluid called latex. This was originally collected from wild trees in South America, but nowadays 90% of rubber production is from the rubber plantations of cultivated trees in Malaysia, Indonesia, Thailand, Sri Lanka and other South East Asian countries. These cultivated trees are the descendents of the seedlings which were germinated at Kew Gardens, London. They were originally grown from the seeds of wild rubber trees obtained in the year 1876 from the lower Amazon basin, in Brazil. Currently the leading natural-rubber-producing countries are Cambodia, China, India, Indonesia, Malaysia, Papua New Guinea, Philippines, Singapore, Sri Lanka, Thailand and Vietnam.

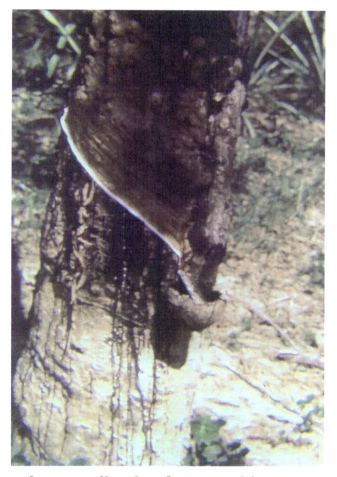

Latex collection from a rubber tree

The latex is collected from the trees by *tapping*. The plantation workers cut a narrow, slanting groove in the trunk just beneath the bark. At the bottom of the cut a metal spout is attached, below which a cup is placed. The milky white latex gradually oozes out from the cut and drips into the cup. In some countries, especially India and Sri Lanka, a half coconut shell is used for collecting the latex.

The latex thus collected contains mainly water (two-thirds); the remaining one-third is the pure rubber. To get rid of the excess water, the collected latex is taken to the plantation factory for processing. The latex can be processed by various methods. One method is to concentrate latex in a centrifuge machine. The machine rotates at high speed and thus flings away the heavier water portion from the rubbery part. The concentrated rubbery part is then preserved by adding ammonia.

Another method is to make crude rubber which is then rolled into sheets so that water is squeezed out. To make the crude rubber, the latex is usually treated with formic acid. Afterwards the rolled sheets are hung in a hot smokehouse for several days. The concentrated latex or rolled rubber sheets (in bales) are then taken to factories for further processing. The dry, raw rubber is made into a soft, pliable, dough-like form by putting it into a machine and heating it, adding a softening agent. The process is called *plasticising*.

40 The next stage of the process is compounding, the object of which is to improve the properties of the rubber by adding fillers (clay), pigments (carbon black) and sulphur. The fillers make the rubber easy to work, pigments increase the strength and durability of the rubber and the sulphur makes it harder, tougher and more elastic.

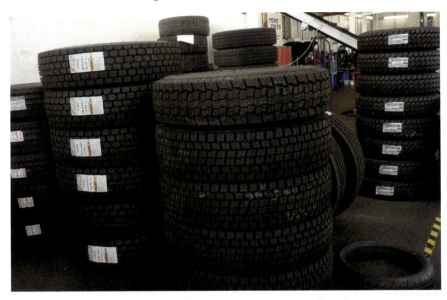

Rubber products – tyres and tubes

Synthetic rubbers are derived from the chemical industry and are man-made products from petroleum. They include styrene-butadiene rubbers, silicone rubbers, butyl rubbers and nitrile rubbers.

Tyres and tubes are the main industrial products from rubber. Various other rubber products are also manufactured for the automotive industry.

Rubber is used in the construction and building industries, mainly for doors, windows, hoses, belts, matting, flooring and dampeners. It also has uses in manufacturing gloves, gum boots, balloons, rubber bands, pencil erasers, adhesive and also in the textile industry. To achieve these products, various manufacturing process are involved in which the rubber is shaped by a variety of methods, such as calendaring, moulding, dipping, vulcanization and so on. Various improved versions of rubber are used in aircraft landing tyres – including space shuttles – and rubber also has its uses for earthquake bearing. Natural rubber materials have always been reused after undergoing a recycling process. Nowadays more use is being made of blends of synthetic and natural rubber.

Since 1988 there has been increased use of natural rubber among health care workers for such things as surgeon's gloves, medical examination gloves, and protective gloves against AIDS, hepatitis etc.

WHAT ARE THE HEALTH ISSUES?

Dust, fume and skin contact are the main health issues. Latex dermatitis is a now well-known phenomenon, as more people are using gloves and more people are reacting to latex. Hence latex rubber allergy is increasing. However there was a debate over who gets the latex allergy: is it more common in the production sector or the consumer sector? It is interesting to note that latex production workers (plantation workers) do not seem to suffer any allergic reactions, despite handling liquid latex in hot, sweaty conditions; on the other hand, health care workers are getting the latex allergy. This may be due to various methods of glove manufacturing using varying levels of protein and powder. Research is in progress to reduce protein levels and develop powder-free coated gloves with improved grip, and to prevent adhering. This may prevent protein allergy problems with the gloves.

The International Agency for Research on Cancer (IARC) Working Group concluded in 1982 that there was sufficient evidence of moderate increase in cancer risks among rubber workers. The risks were for bladder, laryngeal and lung cancer and also for leukaemia. Respiratory and gastro-intestinal mobility are other possible health hazards. Genotoxic hazards cannot be ruled out.

Chapter 18: Sewing

Sewing means fastening or joining various materials using a needle and thread. Cloth, linen, leather, furs and bark are the various materials which are used.

Prior to the introduction of the sewing machine, sewing was done by hand, mostly by females. Archaeological discoveries of bone needles with eyes support the idea that during the Ice Age, bone needles were used to sew animal skins and furs. However, the first workable sewing machine was invented in the year 1790 and since then various attempts have been made to produce a variety of satisfactory workable sewing machines; in 1846 the first automatic sewing machine was invented. In 1851 the Singer machine, with a rigid arm instead of an overhanging one, was introduced for home use.

Traditionally sewing is a female-dominated industry, but some sewing jobs are carried out by male personnel. In some countries children are also employed.

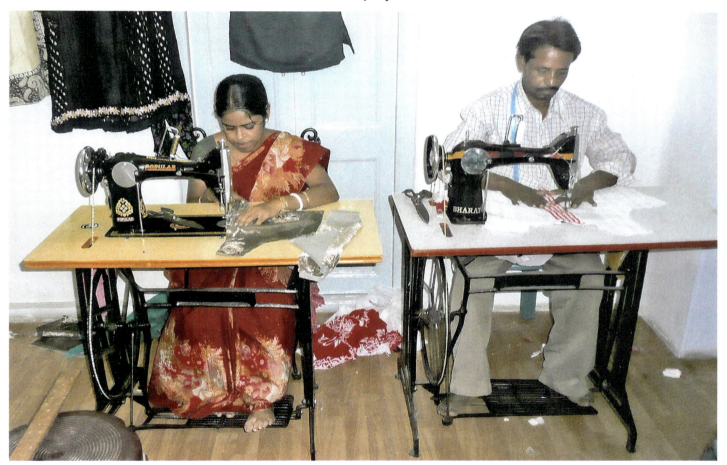

Dressmakers engaged in sewing work (India)

The jobs or occupations which require sewing are dressmaking, tailoring, shoemaking, bookbinding, cloth making, garment making, the manufacture of hats, gloves, bags, suitcases, corsets and quilts, upholstery, taxidermy, parachute and sail making. Upholstery work involves a wide variety of tasks, ranging from domestic and commercial furniture making (sofas, beds, chairs, tables) to the automobile, railway, marine and aviation industries. So it seems that sewing techniques are used in home dressmaking as well as in industries. Seam allowances, sewing tools, accessories and various types of stitches are essential and sometimes soft goods or objects (buckles, buttons, zippers, beads etc.) are sewn into the garments.

42 The sewing tools and accessories are a) pins and needles, made of brass, bronze, steel, bone, antler or silver, b) thimble rings, made of antler, bronze, brass or leather, c) needle tubes, made of antler, brass, bone or wooden, d) awls, made of antler or steel.

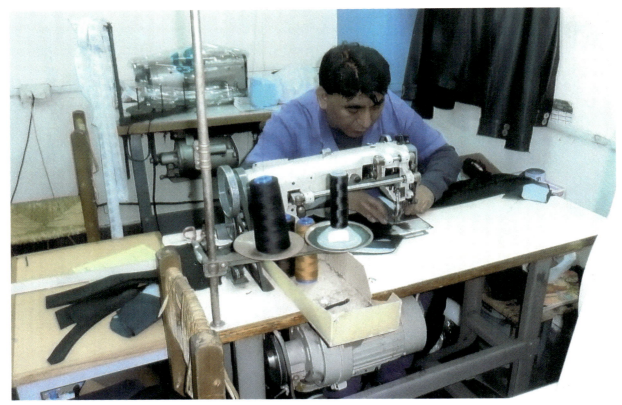

A sewing machinist in Argentina

In machine sewing, to achieve a better class of sewing and avoid any difficulties including health issues, the following factors are to be considered:
a)   correct body posture and correct positioning of the hand so that any kind of awkward posture can be avoided.
b)   good quality needles and thimbles which are not easily breakable.
c)   the correct sizes of hand scissors (one large pair, one small) for various sewing work.
d)   the right type of thread and cut to the correct length.
e)   suitable types of working materials.
f)   comfortable working condition.

Sewing machinists sometimes handle chemicals such as solvents, petroleum products, bleaching products, surfactants, asbestos and cleaning-related products.

WHAT ARE THE HEALTH ISSUES?

Injuries from sharp objects such as needles, pins, scissors and rotary cutters are not uncommon. Posture- and tool-related back and upper limb disorders such as RSI (repetitive strain injury), carpel tunnel syndrome, tendon, elbow and shoulder injuries, and back strain are reported. Eye strain and eye disorders among the operators are also seen and may be worsened by inadequate lighting. Children are more vulnerable. Fabric-related chemical sensitivities can cause lung, skin, liver and kidney lesions. Some of the chemicals are also carcinogenic.

Sugar cane, from which sugar is made, has been an important crop since ancient times. Sugar cane is a kind of herb, belonging to the perennial grass family. It usually grows to a height of 6-24 feet, depending on the species, and has segmented stalks and long pointed leaves. There are barbs at each joint of the segmented stalks, where flowers appear as the plant matures. The plant most probably originated in India and around the Pacific (on the basis of the types of species) and is now grown worldwide. There are between 6 and 37 varieties or species. However, the farmers in India have cultivated sugar cane since ancient times: Alexander's army saw the cane in the fields of India during their conquest in 326 BC. Dioscorides in the first century AD described 'a honey called shakkharon collected from reeds of India'. It was originally grown for chewing because of its high sugar and juice content. The rind was removed by the teeth and the internal contents sucked and chewed. However, crystallised sugar production from cane juice was discovered in India during the Gupta period (320-550 AD), though sugar making by boiling the sugar cane existed in India during the first millennium BC.

Sugar cane is also used as a livestock feed, and has been given to elephants and cattle since ancient times. Sugar cane is still used in the temples of India as a part of ritual offerings to Hindu gods. Sugar cane is now cultivated all over the world and sugar mills produce sugar in most of the regions of the world. Almost 200 countries grow sugar cane now and the top ten countries are Brazil, India, China, Thailand, Pakistan, Mexico, Colombia, Australia, Argentina and the USA.

For planting the seeds are laid horizontally in well-drained soil in rows about 4- 5 feet apart and covered with soil. For optimum growth, fertilisers, herbicides and water irrigation are needed. The cane takes 18-24 months to mature before it is harvested.

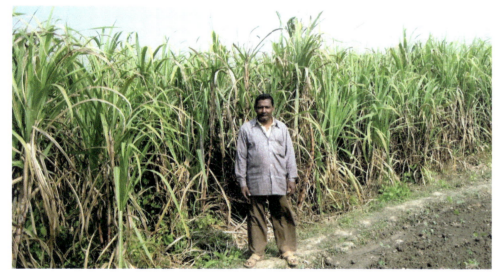

Sugar cane growing in the field

Sugar cane is harvested by hand or mechanically. In hand harvesting, the harvesters cut the cane joints above ground level using cane knives or machetes.

In some countries, such as the USA, when the cane is mature the canes are first burnt in the field, without harming the matured stalks and roots, before the cane is cut. In India, the fields are not burnt before harvesting. After sugar crane is cut, a stem of 0.3 metres is left on the field for further harvest. After 2-3 harvests the whole field is burnt and a new crop is grown: farmers are more dependent on manual activities. In Fiji, the front of the field is usually cleared and prepared for the new crop while the cane at the back is still to be cut. In mechanical harvesting, the modern machine cuts the cane at the base of the stalk, strips the leaves, chops the cane to a consistent length and deposits these canes in the transporter.

Thus, all three activities (reaping, binding and threshing) are done concurrently. From the field, the harvested cane is taken to the mills by various modes of transport; from the primitive (bullock carts, camels) to the modern (vans, lorries, trucks, heavy vehicles or trains).

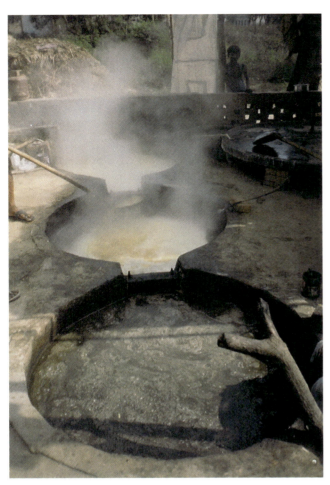

Traditional way of sugar making in India

The cane first goes through the washers and is cut into small pieces and then shredded or crushed. The crushed, macerated cane goes through the rollers, water is added and the sugar juice is taken out, leaving 'bagasse'.

Lime is added to raise the PH and the mixture is heated to 100ºC for several hours. The lime causes suspended materials, proteins, waxes and fats to precipitate. Further impurities are settled in large containers and are removed from the bottom. The residue is known as filter cake or filter mud. The clear juice is again heated in a series of evaporators and separated from the molasses in centrifuges. Here the crystal raw brown sugar is formed, which is further refined and decoloured by centrifuging.

The last stage of the process is the separation, packaging and labelling which is done on the basis of the size of the crystals and the types of sugar i.e. brown or white.

Sugar cane has many other industrial uses. Molasses is a by-product of the manufacturing of cane sugar. This along with cane sugar can be fermented to produce alcoholic drinks such as rum. Ethyl alcohol (ethanol) is also produced from molasses. and this is used in making vinegar, cosmetics, cleaning materials, solvents, coatings and pharmaceuticals.

Ethanol is also a renewable source of fuel for vehicles which is mainly produced in Brazil. In India, sugar cane juice is often prescribed as a therapeutic drink to victims of hepatitis virus infections. The residue left after the juices are extracted is called bagasse and is used for making paper, cardboard, fibre board and wall board. The bagasse is also used as fuel for electrical generators and as cattle feed. Cane wax can be used in the production of polishes and insulation.

WHAT ARE THE HEALTH ISSUES?

Work-related accidents and health problems are quite common in the sugar cane industry. Trips, falls, work-related injuries from sharp objects like knives and slicing machines, conveyor belt accidents and accidents due to gas explosions are the physical hazards. Injuries due to lifting and carrying or to repetitive work, work-posture injuries, health hazards from heat, cold and solar radiation, and accidental burn injuries can also occur. Pesticide-related health impacts on sugar cane farmers have also been reported. Bagassosis is a well-known sugar cane dust disease which affects the lungs of the workers by the inhalation of the dust from dried sugar cane fibres. Increased risk of lung cancer amongst sugar cane farmers and workers is found to be associated with sugar cane exposure.

The tea bush originated where India, China and Myanmar (Burma) meet. However, it was in China that the first tea leaves and plants were successfully cultivated and exported.

The first recorded reference to tea as a medicinal plant dates back to 2737 BC and is by the Chinese author and Emperor Shen Nung. There are many legends and mythology surrounding tea and one of the tea legends is that where Bodhidharma's eyelids fell, the first tea plant grew. Tea is said to be Bodhidharma's gift to the Buddhist world of meditation, as the stimulating effects of tea drinking make tea an aid to alert meditation and spiritual development. In the year 729 AD, along with the Buddhist influence, tea spread to Japan. In the sixth century, it spread to Russia.

In Europe in 1610 AD, the first sample of tea arrived in the Netherlands, although prior to that some tea had reached Europe via the silk route. Later on, Britain became the largest tea market as a tea-drinking nation, and British merchants played an important part in taking it to America and the rest of Europe. In 1823, it was Robert Bruce who rediscovered the tea plant growing in Assam.

The tea plant (*Camellia sinensis*) used to grow widely in Assam; local tribal or aboriginal people used to use it, and in tenth-century Sanskrit literature it is mentioned as a medicinal plant. 1n 1835 the East India Company established tea plantations in Assam.

Nowadays the tea-producing countries are China, India, Sri Lanka, Indonesia, Japan, Taiwan, Bangladesh, Kenya, Uganda, Malawi, Tanzania, Argentina, Brazil, Turkey and Iran.

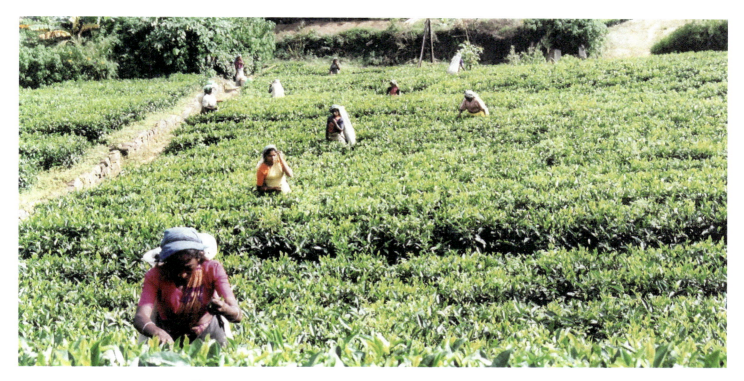

Tea garden and hand tea plucking, Sri Lanka

The suitability of the climate is the important factor in tea growing, as the climate influences yield, crop distribution and quality. Rainfall, temperature, humidity and soil condition are the main issues for the growth of tea bushes. Tea plants grow best on high land with well-drained, fertile acid soil. For good photosynthesis and plant growth, the right length of daylight and the right temperature are vital. The temperature requirement is usually between 10 and 30°C and the annual rainfall requirement is between 1000 and 4000 mm.

In some places, trees are planted to give shade to the bushes; in others wind breaks are placed to prevent damage by strong wind. Tea plants are usually planted in rows and they are kept approximately one metre apart.

The bushes are usually pruned every 2-3 years or 4-5 years depending upon the pruning cycle of the individual tea estate or garden. Usually after 50 years tea plants are replaced by young plants, as by that time the plant's yield is usually reduced. Harvesting fresh young shoots from the mature tea plants is known as plucking: the top 4-5 centimetres are usually picked. Harvesting time is usually throughout the year except winter time; however the best time is from early spring to early summer. Harvesting is usually carried out by women and usually by hand. Tea plucking is an art, as buds and leaves are carefully pinched and twisted when being removed from the tea bush. They are then placed in baskets carried by the pickers on their backs. In some countries, such as Japan, hand picking is replaced by machines and harvest clippers or trimmers are used. After the tea has been harvested from the fields, it is brought directly to the tea factory for further processing.

The traditional method of processing consists of *withering, rolling, oxidation (fermentation) and firing.*
Withering is the first step of tea processing, when freshly harvested tea leaves are spread out on trays or tables so that leaves can air dry. Thus most of the moisture from the leaves is removed. As the moisture evaporates from the leaf, it becomes soft and limp and ready for the next step which is rolling.
Rolling machines break down the cells of the withered leaves, which releases the juices and enzymes from the tea leaves. The rolled leaves are then exposed to air and ready for the next step in the process, which is called *oxidation* or *fermentation.*

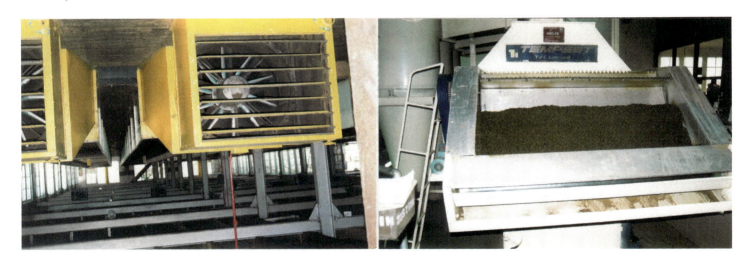

Exhaust and dust cover

For the aroma, flavour and colour of the tea the process of *oxidation or fermentation* is important. As the enzymes and juices in the torn leaves are exposed to air, natural chemical processes take place, giving rise to the distinct aroma or flavour of the tea.
For the colour, the rolled leaves are spread out in a temperature- and humidity-controlled room where the green tea leaves become reddish-brown and then nearly black. The oxidised tea leaves are then taken to a drying chamber, where they are fired or dried by slow heating, and thus the leaves became dehydrated and ready for storage.

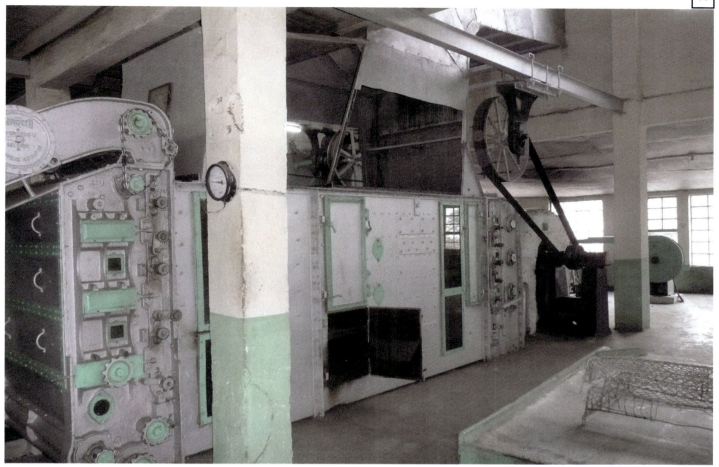

A temperature and humidity control room

Nowadays tea bags are extensively used commercially and for the manufacturing of tea bags the CTC (Cut, Tear, and Curl) processing method is used. The CTC machine cuts, tears and curls the withered tea leaves into a very minute pieces. The leaves are then fired or dried to remove the moisture. The method is quick and in this way a large volume of tea leaves can be processed. Many tea companies now produce tea bags by blending varieties of cut and dried leaf teas from various parts of the world. Once the cut and dried tea leaf is received, it goes for blending and is then sent to tea-packaging machines, where it is packed either as individual tea bags or in bulk packages.

To make instant powder teas, the blended tea requires hot water for brewing. The liquid tea is allowed to concentrate. The concentrated tea spray is dried into a fine powder. It then goes to a package line where it is packed. Sometimes the tea powder is blended with other ingredients, such as sugar or sugar substitute, fruit flavouring or lemon, prior to packaging.

WHAT ARE THE HEALTH ISSUES?

Injuries from burns and accidental injuries due to slipping, tripping and falls can occur. Other issues are noise-induced hearing deficiency, musculo-skeletal (back, arm, shoulders and RSI) disorders, and hand injuries (bruises, lacerations, burns). Skin disorders (dermatitis) and tea-dust-related respiratory disorders are the main health issues. Apart from nuisance dust (coughing and sneezing), persons with chronic bronchitis and asthma run a higher risk of respiratory disorders. Tea-dust related occupational asthma has also been reported.

Index

Acknowledgements

My thanks to those who allowed or arranged my visits or have given permission for the photographs or images that are illustrated in this book with special references to:

1. Rachna Kumar for the Bangles, 2. Jonathan Coate (Basket Maker), P H Coate & Son Ltd. for the willow basket making, 3. Dr Dilip Ghosh for the brick making industry, 4.Jugnu Ray for the embroidery and sewing, 5. Pat Perryman (Allhallows Museum, Honiton) for the Honiton lace making demonstration, 7.Pinaki Mitra for the leather industry, 8.Shyamal Baksi for the plastic industry, and 9. Mrs S Thawani for the crochet lace knitting.

My special thanks also to Dr Rosemary Anne Williams for her help in copy editing, and Stephen Ingarfill for the computing and technical help.

BOOK 2: COMING SOON

It contains the following 20 Chapters:

1. Bee-hive products
2. Card making
3. Comb making
4. Coral and seashell products
5. Cork Making
6. Clock making
7. Doll making
8. Gem stone
9. Jewellery
10. Marble and stone work
11. Mosaics
12. Musical Instruments
13. Salt
14. Spices
15. Tapestry
16. Textile
17. Umbrella making
18. Wood work
19. Whisky making
20. Wine making

BOOK 3: COMING SOON

It contains the following 20 Chapters:

1. Beadwork
2. Beer making
3. Block printing
4. Boat building
5. Cheese-making craft
6. Fireworks
7. Fishing industry
8. Flowers
9. Hydrofoils and Hovercraft
10. Kite making
11. Lock making
12. Paintings
13. Pedicure and Manicure
14. Pearls
15. Potpourri
16. Scaffolding
17. Sculpture
18. Submarine
19. Sholapith craft
20. Totora Reeds work

14068

CPSIA information can be obtained
at www.ICGtesting.com
Printed in the USA
LVIW020553180512

2833LVUK00006B